QUANTITATION IN CARDIOLOGY

BOERHAAVE SERIES
FOR POSTGRADUATE
MEDICAL EDUCATION

PROCEEDINGS OF THE BOERHAAVE COURSES
ORGANIZED BY
THE FACULTY OF MEDICINE, UNIVERSITY OF LEIDEN
THE NETHERLANDS

QUANTITATION
IN
CARDIOLOGY

EDITED BY

H. A. SNELLEN M.D., H. C. HEMKER M.D.,
P. G. HUGENHOLTZ M.D. AND J. H. VAN BEMMEL PH.D.

LEIDEN UNIVERSITY PRESS
1972

SOLE DISTRIBUTOR FOR THE UNITED STATES OF AMERICA AND CANADA
THE WILLIAMS AND WILKINS COMPANY/BALTIMORE

Library of Congress Catalog Card Number 70-188587
ISBN-13:978-94-010-2929-2   e-ISBN-13:978-94-010-2927-8
DOI: 10.1007/978-94-010-2927-8

Jacket design: E. Wijnans gvn

© 1971 Leiden University Press, Leiden, The Netherlands
Softcover reprint of the hardcover 1st edition 1971

CONTENTS

CONCLUDING CHAPTER

CONTRIBUTORS

A. C. Arntzenius, Department of Cardiology, Rotterdam Medical Faculty, Rotterdam, The Netherlands.

C. A. Ascoop, Department of Cardiology, St. Antonius Hospital, Utrecht, The Netherlands.

G. Bell, University Department of Surgery, Royal Infirmary, Glasgow, U.K.

J. H. van Bemmel, Institute of Medical Physics TNO, Utrecht, The Netherlands.

D. L. Brutsaert, Laboratory of Physiology, University of Antwerp, Antwerp, Belgium.

E. Craige, Cardiac Laboratory, North Carolina Memorial Hospital, Chapel Hill (N.C.), U.S.A.

D. Durrer, University Department of Cardiology, Wilhelmina Gasthuis, Amsterdam, The Netherlands.

N. J. Fortuin, Division of Health Effects Research, Department of Medicine, University of North Carolina, Chapel Hill (N.C.), U.S.A.

I. T. Gabe, Royal Postgraduate Medical School, Hammersmith Hospital, London, U.K.

J. Heikkilä, Department of Cardiology, Rotterdam Medical Faculty, Rotterdam, The Netherlands.

P. H. Heintzen, Department of Pediatric Cardiology, University Childrens Hospital, Kiel, West-Germany.

H. C. Hemker, Department of Cardiobiochemistry, University Hospital, Leiden, The Netherlands.

W. Th. Hermens, Department of Cardiobiochemistry, University Hospital, Leiden, The Netherlands.

G. van Herpen, Institute of Medical Physics TNO, Utrecht, The Netherlands

M. R. Hoare, Medical Systems Division, N.V. Philips Gloeilampenfabrieken, Eindhoven, The Netherlands.

L. Hollaar, Department of Cardiobiochemistry, University Hospital, Leiden, The Netherlands.

W. P. Hood, Environmental Protection Agency, Department of Medicine, University of North Carolina, Chapel Hill (N.C.), U.S.A.

P. G. Hugenholtz, Department of Cardiology, Rotterdam Medical Faculty, Rotterdam, The Netherlands.

P. E. Lange, Department of Pediatric Cardiology, University Childrens Hospital, Kiel, West-Germany.

O. A. Larsen, Department of Clinical Physiology, Bispebjerg Hospital, Copenhagen, Denmark.

V. Malerczyk, Department of Pediatric Cardiology, University Childrens Hospital, Kiel, West-Germany.

G. T. Meester, Department of Cardiology, Rotterdam Medical Faculty, Rotterdam, The Netherlands.

C. J. Mills, Royal Postgraduate Medical School, Hammersmith Hospital, London, U.K.

J. M. Neilson, Department of Medical Physics, University of Edinburgh, Edinburgh, U.K.

J. Pilarczyk, Department of Pediatric Cardiology, University Childrens Hospital, Kiel, West-Germany.

J. R. Roelandt, Department of Cardiology, Rotterdam Medical Faculty, Rotterdam, The Netherlands.

H. B. Rubin, Department of Cardiology, University of Southern California, Los Angeles (Cal.), U.S.A.

H. Sandler, NASA-Ames Research Center, Moffet Field (Cal.), U.S.A.

B. McA. Sayers, Engineering in Medicine Laboratory, Imperial College, London, U.K.

W. Schaper, Department of Cardiology, Rotterdam Medical Faculty, Rotterdam, The Netherlands.

R. H. Selvester, Cardiology Service, Rancho de los Amigos Hospital, Downey (Cal.), U.S.A.

L. T. Sheffield, Medical Center, University of Alabama, Birmingham (Ala.), U.S.A.

M. E. Sherman, Air Pollution Control Office, Department of Medicine, University of North Carolina, Chapel Hill (N.C.), U.S.A.

M. L. Simoons, Department of Physiology, University of Utrecht, Utrecht, The Netherlands.

H. A. Snellen, Department of Cardiology, University Hospital, Leiden, The Netherlands.

C. A. Swenne, Institute of Medical Physics TNO, Utrecht, The Netherlands.

B. S. Tabakin, Department of Cardiology, Rotterdam Medical Faculty, Rotterdam, The Netherlands.

C. W. Vellani, Department of Medicine, University of Edinburgh, Edinburgh, U.K.

J. O. Wagner, Department of Medicine, University of Southern California, Los Angeles (Cal.), U.S.A.

S. A. G. J. Witteveen, Department of Cardiobiochemistry, University Hospital, Leiden, The Netherlands.

INTRODUCTORY CHAPTER

INTRODUCTION

This book comprises the essential records from a Boerhaave course given in June 1971 for specialists in cardiology and other fields of internal medicine interested in the subject of quantitation in cardiology. It is evident that in the wide field of medicine, and particularly in cardiology, there is a growing need for exact and detailed information in conjunction with existing diagnostic methods. This is apparent in the greater precision in anatomical and haemodynamic details required by the thoracic surgeon as the number of available heart operations gradually increases. In retrospect it is hardly surprising that the high initial mortality after the introduction of each operation depended to a large extent upon the degree of accuracy with which the diagnosis was made.

Another urgent need for precise and quantitative information became apparent when monitoring of high-risk patients, in order to forestall complications and/or death, became routine. The same applies for the diagnostic procedures used to estimate the patient's chances of surviving an operation and/or rehabilitation after a serious incident, such as myocardial infarction.

In these fields there is a vast amount of data to be handled and – in modern diagnostic procedures – it must be processed so rapidly that the human mind cannot suffice and computer equipment has become indispensable.

These considerations justified a course on quantitative cardiology, the real significance and aim of which are so ably described in Professor Sayers' introductory lecture that elaboration here seems superfluous. We have added some of the discussions to enliven the text, and as an additional source of information.

It should be mentioned that quantitative analysis of the QRS complex in the electrocardiogram and the vectorcardiogram was not included since this was the subject of another international symposium held somewhat later in Amsterdam, 15-16 october 1971, which is also being published.*

* Van Herpen, G., May, J. F., Tuinstra, C. L. & De Vries, T. (eds.), *Automated ECG analyses and its significance for national health care*. Proceedings of a symposium organized by the Dutch Heart Foundation. Den Haag 1972. (In prep.).

3

There are of course other aspects of this vast subject which are not covered in this book, based on a two-day course. However we trust that some of the most important issues have been included. They provided ample food for thought for the participants. We hope that the same will be true for the readers of this book.

H. A. Snellen, H. C. Hemker
P. G. Hugenholtz, J. H. van Bemmel

THE NEED FOR QUANTITATION IN CARDIOLOGY

B. MCA. SAYERS

The progress of science and medicine takes place in various ways. Sometimes a major new advance occurs without being recognized at all, and then, after the event, it is discovered that a great change in mental processes and attitudes has taken place quite spontaneously. But sometimes there is a conjunction of circumstances, and it is possible for the careful observer to recognize that some new approach in medicine is now due, and that the development of the scientific or technological capability to make a new advance possible is now imminent. On the whole, to recognize such a conjunction or any other sign of a notable imminent advance, we have no option but to apply our best endeavours to evaluate the likely long-term value and consequences of the possibilities that come on to our horizons.

One of these possibilities could now be on the horizon – in fact, it is possible that we may now be seeing early signs (straws in the wind) that a new kind of quantitative medicine, not just a new and more quantitative phase of medicine, is on its way. We can be sure that any such eventuality would greatly influence cardio-respiratory medicine in general and cardiology in particular. So it is worthwhile to try to look forward and to imagine likely developments in quantitative medicine to assess if their impact on cardiology and other aspects of medicine will be widespread, potent and fundamentally important – and if, therefore, the present signs do indeed herald an imminent major advance.

Before we start in on this task, it is good to remind ourselves of the difficulty of projecting ourselves outside our immediate intellectual and mental framework, either to look to the past, or to the future. Looking backwards to the great advances of the past, it is almost impossible to comprehend the brilliance of achievement of many great medical and scientific workers, simply because we cannot free ourselves from our present insights. Similarly it is very hard to look forward – to imagine in any concrete way what developments are going to affect our professional activities, the way we think about them, and the way we carry them out. We are constrained between the influence of our recent years and our present insights. Furthermore it is even much easier to anticipate a new development than to know where it is leading.

It is from this position of difficulty (bearing in mind the straws in the wind that we may be able to identify) that we are meeting here to consider one of the ideas in our own field that might possibly greatly affect the cardiologist from now on, that might possibly alter greatly the way he carries on his cardiology and the way he thinks about it. We are meeting to consider an idea, the idea of a quantitative cardiology, whose time might possibly be imminent.

Some extensive quantitation in cardiology is now possible and very much more is now obviously feasible but not yet turned into reality. But, is the idea of a new and extensive quantitation in cardiology one of these powerful, worthwhile, unavoidable developments? It is only possible to come to a decision about this by focussing on specific issues and a few of these are central.

The essential questions are these:

1. Can we achieve stable, reliable and reproducible quantitative results in a range of cardiological measurement?
2. Given that accurate quantitative measurements can be made under clinical conditions can we positively interpret the results in terms of the patient's bodily processes?
3. Given accurate measurements, adequately related to physiological and pathological facts and events, can these be integrated into a coherent and quantitative assembly of facts from which new insight can be gained into the clinical condition of the patient, into trends in clinical condition, and to provide indications of impending catastrophes?
4. Given that new diagnostic or clinical insight can be achieved, is it possible to use the particular kind of insight that can be reached in this way in order to provide concrete guidance in taking serious therapeutic decisions?

Now, it obviously does matter if the quantitative magnitude of cardiac output in a given patient is say, 4.5 l/min, provided of course that we have a point of reference – such as the information that 48 hours previously the figures was say, 5.5 l/min. And in general, I think we can take it that getting a new and better series of numbers to extend the description of cardiac function in the patient is certainly now possible and this meeting will cover many of these. Developments in stable and reliable measurement are indeed being achieved. But if that were all this would be just another worthwhile but typical advance in the subject which would lead us only a limited distance. On the other hand, it is my speculation that what will emerge is an approach to cardiology which will allow us to interpret the measurements in detail – more especially in the context of the overall set of interacting control systems with which the heart and circulation are involved. This goes for the control of blood pressure, of blood chemistry, of respiratory gas exchange and of myocardial work; it goes also for the underlying drive to maintain adequate tissue perfusion by establishing collateral pathways in the coronary circulation, as well as for biochemical control action, and so on. I cannot deny that this is likely to be quite complex but I am sure that as knowledge advances step by step we will be able to make use of each new step of understanding in a highly practical way – provided that the right approach is taken.

This kind of attack will entail measurements of a rather different kind, or more accurately, measurements analysed and interpreted in a rather different way from what has been previously possible. The aim is of course, still the same – to come to an integrated picture of the state of the heart and circulation and its capacity to accept the challenges due to mechanical demands originating in the body's metabolic needs or due to trauma or pathological conditions. Furthermore in the acute patient, we are interested in changes and trends in mechanical and biochemical factors and their influence on clinical condition, and in achieving early warning of impending disasters. In my view the answers to all these specific possibilities as posed above, are becoming increasingly positive. And the final question – about utilizing the results of quantitative manipulation of clinical observations for clinical purposes – yet remains to be attacked in detail.

Returning now to consider fundamentals, the implication underlying the questions raised here is that the traditional representation of facts about the patient can, and perhaps should, be supplemented by a different representation – depending on quantitative details and leading to a quantitative description. This claim would certainly be true if it could be shown that there are aspects of clinical patho-physiology, the understanding of which is now within grasp, that need interpretation in terms of numbers, and that are relevant to clinical purposes.

In my view this is exactly the situation. As soon as we allow ourselves the opportunity to take extensive measurements from the patient to guide therapy, the possibility of greatly enhanced clinical insight arises, provided that the observations can be interpreted. For this purpose it is important to take account of the body control systems mainly involved, their mode of operation, and their reserve capability, and such matters can only be handled

by a strictly quantitative approach. I hope to show that important discrimin-
ations between alternative possibilities depend upon the way the numbers
come out. While it needs to be remembered that the final decision about the
patient on the basis of the observations may still be a dichotomous 'yes – no'
choice, nevertheless in many significant situations we need quantitative
manipulation of quantitative observations to get us to this point of judgement. And this matter raises perhaps the most important meaning of quantitation in medicine – the application of quantitative methods of thought to the
simplification and interpretation of complex clinical observations.

I would explain the matter in this way. Many control systems exist in the
body to regulate levels (of temperature, hormone concentration, blood
pressure and so on) or to manage chemical or physical processes (in terms
of energy cost, power level and reserve capability – as for example, with the
processes of internal and external respiration). These systems clearly exist to
protect against disturbances, most obviously of course due to external factors, but equally due to internal perturbations, including those due to
aberrant behaviour or defects of elements of the system. Consequently in
disease or trauma, relevant control systems in the body must certainly still
be assumed operative, perhaps working vigorously to compensate for pathological effects. I think we must presume that it will become increasingly important to ensure that the therapy co-operates with, or at least does not operate antagonistically to, the compensating operations of natural control
systems. This means, *inter alia*, that we need to know the nature and structure
of the control system, its essential mode of operation, its operating point
(how close to complete breakdown of compensation this system is), both
normally, and in the current circumstances, which in the clinical situation
may be pathological. These are no easy requirements. Even if the system is
known in adequate detail in the normal individual, the trauma or pathology
may have sufficiently altered system elements that its structure is, in effect,
significantly different from that in the normal. Equally, its dominant mode
of behaviour may be quite different.

For these reasons, an evaluation of at least some body control systems
must certainly be expected to become part of the armoury of the clinician
in the near future, and some appreciation of what is involved is likely to pay
clinical dividends immediately. And this is where we become involved in
quantitation. In probing and assessing control systems of the kind met in
physiology, quantitative methods cannot be avoided.

Illustrating this point we can proceed at various levels of complexity.
First, I will show that quantitative detail is relevant to understanding body

dynamic control mechanisms in the body and I will comment on their clinical relevance. Second, the mode of operation of such systems will be shown subject to change in various circumstances, and the task of identifying and interpreting the mode will certainly depend on quantitative methods. Third, I hope to illustrate the way in which quantitative methods of analysis open up typical quantitative measurements as sources of considerable, perhaps unsuspected, further information beyond what is superficially obvious. Fourth, I will outline an example showing how a quantitative style of thought leads to proposals for a firm attack on a difficult, seemingly unspecific, problem of detecting and evaluating trends in clinical condition of the acutely ill patient. Finally, I intend to discuss briefly the kind of suggestions for clinical application raised by quantitative ways of thinking about clinical physiology. It is the intention that the detailed discussions that now follow will not only illustrate the basic point, but also illuminate more general issues.

I start the elaboration of these points by illustrating the need for a quantitative approach in interpreting control system behaviour and by explaining how a quantitative approach provides a framework in which we can gain further insight into the origin and meaning of the observations we can make on the cardiovascular system, especially in relation to the feedback control systems that are involved. While I choose a simple example to illustrate the point, the kind of matter I describe is quite general and enormously important. And in the example I quote, you will be able to see that the simple framework we set up out of our quantitative analysis, does indeed allow us to gain much enhanced insight into cardiac function and the behaviour of the CV system, including the regulating control systems that greatly influence cardiac activity.

The specific example is the pressor system involving baro-receptors in the carotid sinus and aortic arch. The reflexes concerned have the essential task to regulate mean arterial blood pressure and sufficient is known about this system for us to put together its essential elements. It makes up one of the major feedback systems in which cardiac function is directly implicated.

Start with the mean arterial blood pressure and assume constant cardiac output. Imagine that, for some unspecified reason, the pressure falls slightly. The pressure receptors in the carotid sinus and aortic arch alter their firing rate and hence the afferent input to the brain stem. Increased sympathetic outflow results and the smooth muscle of the peripheral blood vessels responds with a vaso-constriction that increases the blood pressure, so compensating the original drop in pressure. Certainly there are other effects including venomotor and inotropic responses, but focussing on this particular reflex, those facts are correct and the kind of description I have given can be found in many modern text-books of medical physiology; we have simply put together a series of elements, or blocks, of a feedback system and the pictorial result would be a block diagram of the system.

But, while the separate elements exist and the steps outlined are probably beyond question, the overall picture is totally insufficient and quite misleading; the system does not behave as simply as that. To interpret the system I need more quantitative details. And when I look all the way round the system in a quantitative way, I find that the numbers tell me something different from the result of a simple inspection of the block diagram.

Assume that all the quantitative data is available and we re-explore the matter. Imagine a small, brief, disturbance imposed on the arterial pressure. The way such a disturbance is handled depends very largely on the detailed quantitative nature of the smooth muscle response; slow disturbances would be handled much as I have described already, but fast disturbances are treated very differently in that, usually, the compensating reaction in pressure returned to the original point of disturbance is quite similar to the original disturbance, and, quantitatively, at least as large.

The compensating reaction produces a response which can totally take the place of the initial disturbance, even if the latter is complete and finished. And what happens then? To keep the story short, the whole system oscillates, and therefore produces a spontaneous, broadly periodic, fluctuation of pressure with a period which can be calculated to be about 10 seconds.

Now we can consider relevant observations in man. These broadly periodic oscillations can indeed be seen clearly in intra-arterial pressure recordings. Additionally, similar components exist in heart rate, as we could expect from the existence of a pathway effectively from brain stem to the sino-atrial node, although I should mention that some different effects also contribute to the way in which the vasomotor system affects heart rate. But it should be very evident from this example that the properties of biological control systems do indeed require quantitative interpretation; a semantic, or non-quantitative, description will not serve.

There is a further, rather strange, aspect of this blood pressure behaviour which cannot be understood without careful attention to the quantitative properties of the control system. This system has two modes of behaviour. Understanding this behaviour and identifying the mode of operation needs quantitative analysis.

The matter arises because the brain-stem afferent-efferent interface has the property, in essence, of responding in on-off fashion. Pressures generally below a certain level generate almost full magnitude responses, while pressures above this level produce no sympathetic outflow. As a result certain kinds of external disturbance imposed on the system will affect its behaviour in the following way. If the external disturbance is very roughly periodic, the effect is to reduce the magnitude of any compensating reaction to blood pressure fluctuations, indeed perhaps to the point where the spontaneous oscillations of the system cannot be sustained. In this situation the only fluctuations of the system are those which are periodic with a period equal to that of the external disturbance and this effect is known as entrainment. It is made possible because the external disturbance can have the effect of reducing the magnitude of intrinsic reactions to pressure fluctuations initiated within the system, and this reduction is in turn made possible because of the brain-stem properties.

For external disturbances of small magnitude or low periodic frequency, the interference between external disturbance and system properties may be insufficient to stop the spontaneous oscillation; then the mean blood pressure signal shows both fluctuations. Carrying out a detailed numerical analysis of the system, it appears that if the external, broadly periodic, disturbance is low frequency (that is, long period), entrainment is very difficult to achieve, and can only be achieved at all with large magnitudes of the disturbance. But if the disturbance frequency is near or above the frequency of spontaneous oscillation, entrainment can be achieved easily even with small magnitude disturbances.

So we have a frequency-selective effect in entrainment, which we call, briefly, selective-entrainment. And in the practical cardiovascular system, in man, we can readily see this effect happening – because respiration serves as an effective external disturbance of a broadly periodic kind. Spontaneous oscillations of the kind I have mentioned, vaso-motor oscillations, with about a 10-second period in man, can be selectively entrained by respiration. It is possible to see, often very clearly, the onset of spontaneous oscillation and its entrainment in, say, the heart rate, or arterial blood pressure. So the system has two modes of behaviour – oscillatory and non-oscillatory – and I must point out that once this is recognized, interpretation of this aspect of blood pressure (or heart rate) is fairly simple, but without any such recognition the behaviour of the system inevitably appears complicated and indeed confusing.

Incidentally another very similar system also contributes to the blood pressure and heart rate behaviour. Again by a careful quantitative analysis it is possible to show that the first line of thermal defence in the body is based on a regulating system that involves superficial blood vessels, hypothalamic- and skin-temperature receptors, and the vaso-motor system. This system is also strongly non-linear, and oscillates spontaneously but in a more compli- cated way; since it influences blood flow it produces an effect on the baro-re- ceptors, and so contributes a very slow disturbance not only to the blood pressure systems, but also to heart rate (1).

So here we have two body control systems, that happen to influence the cardiovascular system in a way which affects certain physiological variables commonly recorded for clinical purposes; both show rather peculiar prop- erties, both need to be interpreted in a quantitative way, and both de- monstrate modes of behaviour that can only be recognized by quantitative analysis of the measurements that can be made.

Now that the basic features of these systems have been identified, the quantitative methods required to identify the state of the system say, are well-defined and fairly simple to use. But, despite the fact that these methods are simple, they cannot be dispensed with; quantitation in still essential. It cannot be overlooked that what is true of these systems is likely also to be true of many others in the body, especially the major endocrine systems that are so complex to understand at present; hence, an insight, necessarily quantitative, into the nature and behaviour of body control systems in general must be of great clinical significance in the near future. But it is possible to come to immediate practicalities; the integrity and capability of the cardiovascular control systems are clearly of utmost interest in the cardiac medical or surgical patient and these may be evaluated by probing the system – applying a small test stress and observing the system response, in delay, magnitude and form.

The cardiovascular system includes several obviously interacting feedback systems. Demands placed on one of these react on the others and it is vital to remember that systems whose function is to regulate some internal environ- mental factor will often do so (with support from the other systems) fairly effectively even though the system, or the demand on it, is pathological in the extreme. This is the reason why we need to assess the reserve, and the cost to the system in meeting existing demands, rather than simply how well the arterial pressure and stroke volume is maintained. Bushman, working at the Royal College of Surgeons of England, has already been developing such an evaluation, by imposing a kind of Valsalva manoeuvre and measuring both the immediate response and the result of restoring normal intrathoracic pressure.

This is one of a number of possible dynamic tests that make use of quantitative methods in interpreting, for strictly immediate clinical purposes, the reserve capability and current state of the cardiovascular regulating system.

In each case the task is inevitably quantitative tactically, and has a strategically important aim – to attempt to predict the future capability of the system under examination, and to decide how it should be supported if this is needed. And it is with this kind of aim in mind that I have illustrated with my previous examples that at least the first steps can be taken in identifying some of the interacting control systems and their behaviour, whether they are neural, biochemical, mechanical or physiological.

Next I would like to turn to the application of quantitative methods to analysis of appropriate physiological measurement; in short, this shows that such signals may contain information much beyond what is superficially obvious. Even in the case of the heart rate or cardiac interbeat interval signal, judicious analysis by quantitative methods (mainly by techniques of digital filtering utilizing a digital computer) allows a reasonable resolution of a number of different influences – due to respiration, vasomotor activity involved in the regulation of blood pressure, vasomotor activity due to skin temperature gradient control for preservation of core temperature, together with changes imposed by circulatory redistributions, and mental work load (2). Not all of these influences can be effectively described in quantitative fashion by separating out the relevant contribution in the heart rate signal but some undoubtedly can, and in any case indications are often available of significant alterations in various originating processes due to physiological changes, including those of pathological origin (3). I am sure that it will become clear as the meeting proceeds that as soon as steps are taken to make continuing quantitative observations in cardiology, a signal becomes available that is amenable to detailed scrutiny by quantitative methods, often leading to much potentially valuable information which can indicate or describe the state of the patient or the current mode of behaviour of some of his underlying systems.

The various examples I have quoted so far are rudimentary but I hope they do illustrate the potential strategic importance of quantitative methods in practical clinical medicine. What I have tried to do is to put a little flesh on the bones of an idea – that there is something far-reaching about the quantitative approach to medicine in general, and cardiology in particular. In a nutshell: the quantitative strategy is a frame of mind – that seeks for insight into the relation between, on the one hand, the dynamics of the physiological variables and clinical signs, and on the other, the clinical condition of the patient. This frame of mind allows us to recognize that a pictorial description of the complex, interacting set of incompletely compensating systems that is the patient, simply will not do; we cannot avoid a detailed quantitative description if we are to understand what is happening – we cannot do without the numbers.

The poet Coleridge remarked that 'men must be weighed, not counted,' and, despite an apparent pre-occupation with numbers, we need to recognize, equally, that the whole purpose of our quantitative activities is to allow us to weigh the implications of what we are seeing, or counting, or calculating. Just because many of us are tied up with tactics in the computer operations we rely on for our data processing, does not mean we do not have a strategy – a means of searching for the implication of the results we obtain from our tactical operations. I myself have been inevitably much concerned with detailed tactics in several different kinds of analysis of records from acute cardiac patients in the Intensive Care situation; but the strategy is very clear. Changes and trends in clinical condition of the patient must be detected. I might wish to determine from the physiological measurements if the apparently uncomplicated recovery of, for example, one particular patient is masking an incipient deterioration. In another case I might wish to know if the patient is showing any early indications of developing arrythmia. In yet another case I may wish to establish if the patient is making reasonable progress at the expense of long term integrity of his myocardium, or of his coronary blood supply and so on. It must not be thought these questions can all be answered; nevertheless, some preliminary schemes are becoming available for weighing up the significance of results, and again, quantitative methods are required to put the results of first-stage processing into a form allowing decisions to be made.

The essence of the tactical matter is quickly stated: quantitative, numerical, methods are important for manipulating the measurements – that is, for processing. Most of the measurements we can make directly, are not usable directly for the purposes we have in mind. Processing is required. Indeed in all the examples I have referred to already, numerical processing of the record is essential – to extract the numbers we want (such as the intervals between successive heart beats), to suppress unwanted information, to highlight significant features of the record, and to allow us to identify the ebb and flow of the components of interest. These (so called, first-stage operations) are all numerical operations, performed on the raw signal that comes from the patient, by special purpose electronic apparatus, or nowadays, mainly by computer – that can be set up to behave like any special purpose apparatus.

The strategic matter is more far-reaching; because almost no attention has been hitherto given to quantitative methods for studying trends in clinical condition by investigating alterations appearing in physiological records, I will discuss this matter in somewhat more detail. The techniques involved are those that might give indications if the clinical progress of the patient is uneventful and substantially free of complications, or if the patient's progress is likely to be complicated by undesirable developments. In the case of the patient with acute coronary heart disease, the complications concerned are those of severe arrythmia or deterioration of myocardial condition. In severe myocardial infarction the electrocardiogram is commonly abnormal in shape. As the patient recovers, this shape abnormality alters somewhat and, broadly speaking, in a generally consistent fashion as time passes. And, of course, in the presence of occasional arrythmias, the basic pattern of the electrocardiogram also tends to fluctuate. Indications are that there are, superimposed on the basic change of shape of the ECG, transient alterations that seem to precede the appearance of a ventricular ectopic focus (3). Unhappily, to see these transient changes clearly, it is necessary to emphasize the highfrequency part (the rapid events) of the ECG (and this produces some inconvenience, as well as greatly changing the signal shape). Consequently it is useful to utilize the high-frequency (HF) ECG as a basic signal for trend detection purposes. However other signals are also available and may be more useful in some circumstances.

Consider then the behaviour of HF ECG following, say, acute myocardial infarction; in addition to short duration transient effects over periods of hours, there is a general change with the passage of time as the patient recovers, or otherwise. Now when such a continuous change is going on, it is worthwhile to ask about the underlying process causing the change – in particular, to ask if the process is essentially stable, or if it is fluctuating in a manner which may warn of cardiac arrhythmias or other changes. But there can be a serious difficulty here because if we consider three representative waveforms A, B, C (recorded at 24 hour intervals say) it is often impossible to determine by inspection if the process that altered the pattern A to pattern B, is the same kind of process that altered the pattern B to pattern C. The reason is that the reference patterns (A in one case, B in next) are different. Yet precisely this question is central to identifying consistent trends in clinical condition from physiological, biochemical, or other observations, so an answer is needed to the problem. And it seems to be available.

The scheme I describe here is only one of a class of schemes, but it is very simple and involves few special procedures. It works as illustrated in figure 1.

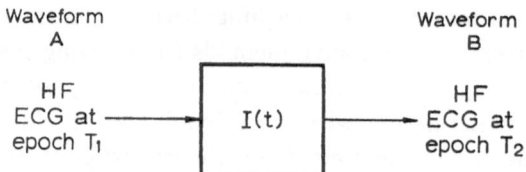

I(t) specifies impulse response of required linear system

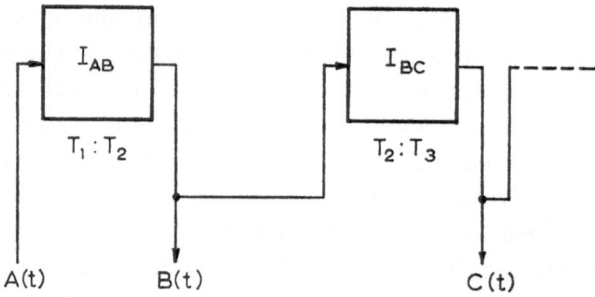

Fig. I. Trend function analysis applied to the high frequency electrocardiogram. Recordings at T_1 and T_2 are compared and the impulse response of the linear system that will transform waveform A, recorded at epoch T_1, into the second waveform, B, recorded at epoch T_2, is calculated. The lower diagram shows how successive trend functions, relating A with B, B with C, and so on, are determined. The shape of the functions I_{AB}, and I_{BC} are compared to identify the presence or absence of consistent trends as indicated by, in this case, the electrocardiogram.

Waveforms A and B are those (HF ECG patterns in this case) recorded at (say) a 24-hour interval (times T_1 and T_2); A is treated as the input to a linear network, B is treated as the output, and the characteristic of the network that would transform A to B is determined. For this purpose the most convenient network characteristics is its impulse response: the output generated by the network in response to a narrow pulse applied at the input – a description that fully represents the network in all operational respects. For the present I am referring to this description as a trend function, which can be calculated repeatedly for the successive pairs of waveforms produced as time passes; similarities between these successive trend functions indicate a steady trend in patient's condition, as reflected in the waveform of the HF ECG. When no change occurs between successive waveforms, so that A and B are identical, the impulse response becomes simply a narrow spike so it is very easy to recognize. This method puts the changes in the physiological record under study on a footing that allows them to be compared quite readily with changes occurring at earlier or later stages of therapy, and in principle, can be applied to any biological signal, not just the ECG. Indeed this approach can be extended to the 2-dimensional trend-function description necessary to take account of simultaneous changes in two separate signals. (I should remark that there are some technical traps for the unwary in evaluating these functions. Furthermore, if the duration of the QRS contribution to the HF ECG alters, spectral shifts follow; the easiest device that seems satisfactory pragmatically, is to work with smoothed spectral components, averaging neighbouring spectral terms.)

It is instructive to consider what manner of quantitative representation is necessary to describe the process underlying the change between waveforms; some insight into what is required will clarify the choice of trend function described above. If the state of the myocardium alters, locally or more globally, (for example due to changes in local blood supply, or local biochemistry, for pathological reasons) local alterations in electrical excitability will occur, and this must modify the depolarization propagation process. Hence the route of the wave of depolarization through the ventricular tissue must be expected to change, and when this happens, the contribution to the overall electrical activity due to events in any given small region may appear at a different relative time in the electrical waveform. Consequently any function description of the change must have the capability to accommodate this 'time-shuffling', as it were, as well as the altered magnitude of some contributions. (This is why simple differences cannot generally be used to describe such changes.) Put another way, the hypothetical network we are inventing, having the capability to transform one waveform, A, to another, B, must be able to store some component elements that occur at a given time in A, and reproduce them at a different time, for waveform B. On the other hand, since no practicable picture is available, at least in the context of routine analysis, of the minutae of the elemental contributions to the overall electrocardiogram from different small regions in the heart, only an average description of this time-shuffling of contributions can be achieved. Nevertheless, incorporating all these features and requirements into a mechanism to transform one waveform into another (and this is a technical signal handling task), we are immediately led to prescribe a linear network, (the descriptive function of which is its impulse response) because the way in which such a network operates on an input waveform to produce an output (see figure 1) precisely reproduces the above outline of operations required. So, given waveforms A and B, the corresponding network impulse response purports to

describe the physiological process of change. Hence there is a rational basis
for the trial of this kind of trend function, but of course other schemes may
be more productive in practice and I would certainly hope to stimulate
thought about this kind of potential advance.

The essence of the whole idea is to achieve a compact, easily interpreted,
basis for utilizing physiological or biochemical alterations during the course
of therapy, to provide any further insight that might be possible into trends
in the patient's condition; the methods concerned are inevitably quantitative
and as experience of this or similar schemes increases further quantitative
evaluation of the results should certainly lead to a further advance – provided
that it proves sensible in the long run to think about existence of consistent
trends in clinical conditions, rather than of sequences of physiological or
biochemical activity initiated by triggering events. This issue remains to be
resolved but it does seem very clear that both types of behaviour must be
anticipated; even within the context of acute coronary heart disease there
seems to be little doubt that, superimposed on a steady change, transient
changes occur that are presumably initiated by what can be operationally
defined as trigger events. In any case present experience points in this direction and it is appropriate at this stage to illustrate briefly the typical findings.

Figure 2 shows a sequence of trend functions, broadly covering a period
of several days during which the patient made a wholly uneventful recovery
from myocardial infarction. The sequence is typical amongst our results so
far, and it is worth noting the steady approach towards a single spike (so-
called Dirac pulse) form of function indicating, at that stage, little shape
change in the successive HF ECG complexes. The case in which complications
develop seems to produce a very different sequence of trend functions, as
illustrated in figure 3. The differences are very obvious and should provide a
means for following clinical progress at least in one respect, i.e., as evidenced
by the behaviour of the variable studied. In the first instance, the question
which may be adequately answered in this way is if the changes seen at one
stage are consistent with changes seen at an earlier stage; certainly the present indications are that the present method or some equivalent other scheme,
will provide the necessary answers at least in some cases, but further positive
information must still be expected from satisfactory trend function schemes.

Various possibilities of a similar kind exist for quantitative analysis of this
type applied to other signals, not only those of electrocardiographic type;
furthermore, there are advantages, in some circumstances, in working with a
scheme that allows the trend function to represent a specific kind of non-
linear operation. But it must be emphasized that in this type of work, the

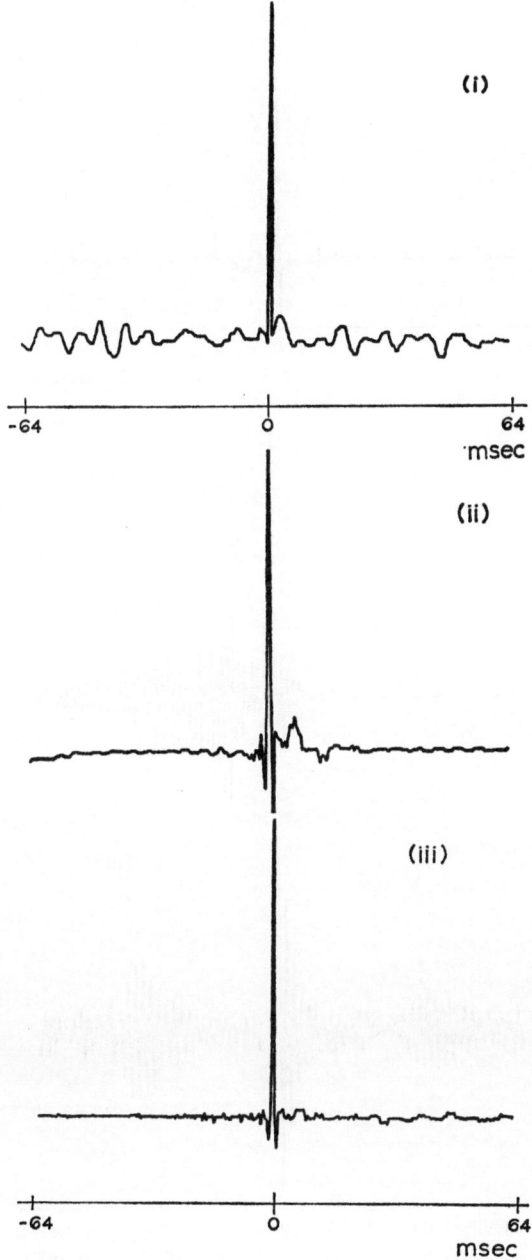

Fig. 2. Three trend functions, based on comparisons at 24 hour intervals on three occasions after hospitalisation, for a patient with acute myocardial infarction; recovery was wholly uneventful.

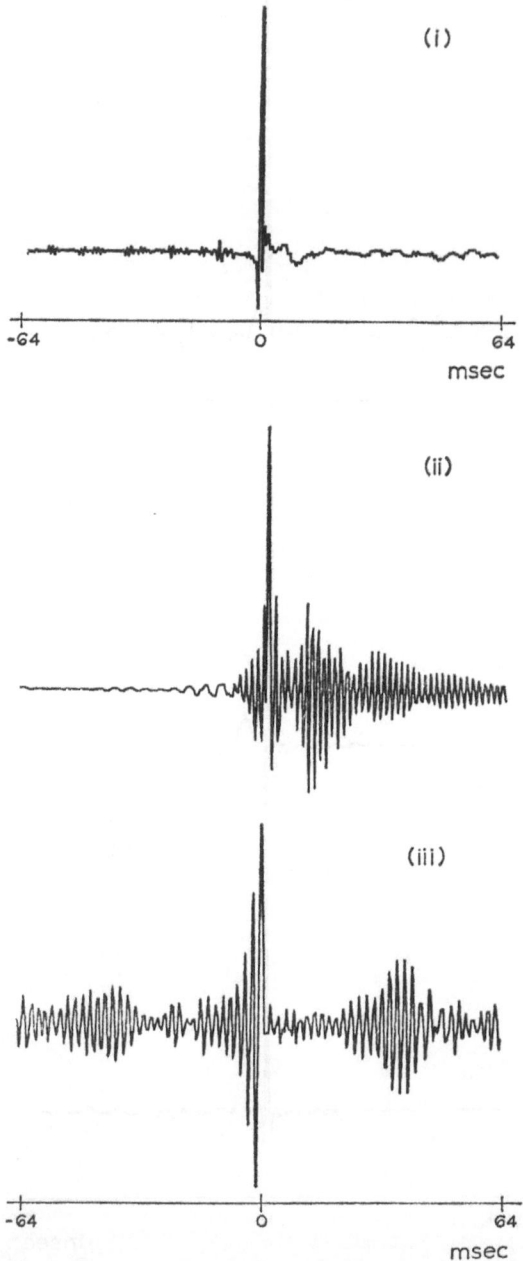

Fig. 3. Three trend functions, as in figure 2, for a similar patient who developed severe arrhythmias, exhibiting ultimately ventricular ectopic events, and subsequent to the period shown here, ventricular fibrillation.

tactics are wholly subsidiary to the strategic purpose of leading to deeper insight into the changes in condition of the patient. Equally, of course, for this purpose we cannot do without the tactics of computer manipulation of the raw signals.

In my view, the example puts the situation in a nutshell. Here we have a technique, an extrapolation from the evidence, that might give indications if the electrocardiographic changes are consistent with a picture of the patient's continuing uncomplicated recovery, or not. There would seem to be no simpler alternatives to this procedure which therefore offers a potential advance in clinical insight with all that implies. And, of course, to match this technique there are, and must be, many others, related to other aspects of cardiological measurements and study. So, computer manipulation of quantitative data in cardiology therefore does obviously have the potential of offering new possibilities for clinical insight and allowing the patient's progress to be subject to much closer surveillance and ultimately, much closer control.

Consequently it is now both sensible and timely to think about putting together the methods of measurement, the techniques of analysis, and the requirements of the clinician, to see how to investigate more closely the state and needs of the patient. This undoubtedly requires the existence of an enlarged group of informed clinical workers who are able to enter into the spirit of these endeavours. It is already clear, and will be further demonstrated by later presentations at this meeting, that the traditional representation of facts about the patient can now certainly be supplemented by new representations, selectively emphasizing various, perhaps newly-clarified, matters. Consequently, if the cardiologist can recruit reasonable flexibility of mind to make use of these new representations (which after all can be aimed to present information selectively in a way which is specially well suited to human mental processes) he could initiate a most significant advance.

In summary then, nearly all our quantitative activities are designed to provide new, clarified, or enhanced information about the diagnostic or clinical state of the patient in detail, the presence of slow trends, and to warn of imminent changes; also some of the developments we must anticipate will present this information in a broader context of the action of underlying and interacting physiological and biochemical regulating processes. Thus, what is now needed in the current climate of developments is to determine how the results can best be used to guide the therapy. This is where the clinician can become closely interested and involved, especially if he appreciates the tactical and strategic purposes behind the quantitative techniques he is offered.

And this raises the question of specific clinical applications which is the focus of this meeting. It is clear from the literature that many exist and the presentations here will have much to report about clinical applications of various quantitative methods. But it is helpful to remember one or two points relating to quantitation, in studying these presentations. Most of the techniques lead to numerical results from which, it is hoped, a clinical decision can be made about therapy or prognosis, but some utilize quantitative methods operating on quantitative observations to lead to results that need not be explicitly numerical but from which, as before, a clinical judgement can be achieved. Some of the presentations refer in detail to studies of physiological mechanisms under normal and pathological conditions; others, like quantitative graded exercise testing, will be concerned with methods of probing the feedback system involved in cardiovascular response to load, and with methods of analysing and interpreting results. And in all of the presentations, explicitly stated or implicit, there are clear indications of the vital importance, especially for cardiology, of the reactions of interacting feedback control systems.

Undoubtedly we are at an early stage of understanding. But to make progress here, either in the personal sense or in global terms of medical knowledge generally, there is no substitute for the continuing practical trial of quantitative ideas and quantitative interpretation. I discussed at some length earlier the idea that even some of the simplest clinical measurements that can be made undoubtedly do carry information about detailed physiological activity, to an extent that is totally unrevealed by the usual superficial inspection of the record. It is, indeed, probably profitable to take up the position that this is possibly true of virtually all the quantitative observations one can make in a clinical context; furthermore, it is probably equally profitable to presume that dynamic physiological or biochemical measurements reflect the action of underlying control systems, perhaps of considerable complexity, but at least likely to show dominant characteristics of behaviour which can be identified, and once identified, utilized subsequently for evaluating physiological behaviour. I would remark that taking up the frame of mind which looks at the measurements in this way is in itself an important scientific step and a predisposition to advancing insight. And this is, after all, precisely the aim of advancing quantitation in cardiology.

REFERENCES

1. Hyndman, B. W., Kitney, R. I. & Sayers, B. McA., Spontaneous rhythms in physiological control. *Nature* 233, 339-341 (1971).

2. Sayers, B. McA., The analysis of cardiac interbeat interval sequences. *Proc. roy. Soc. Med.* 64, 707-710 (1971).

3. Sayers, B. McA., *The exploitation of biological signals.* Inaugural lecture, Imperial College, Jan. 26, 1970.

CHAPTER I

MYOCARDIAL INFARCTION

QUANTITATIVE DIAGNOSIS OF
MYOCARDIAL INFARCTION

D. DURRER

A quantitative diagnosis of myocardial infarction in clinical electrocardiography is the accurate prediction of location, size and degree of intramural extension of the infarcted area. This is only possible if several conditions are fulfilled.

1. The QRS-T-changes of myocardial infarction, either acute or chronic, should be specific; their presence should be equivalent to the existence of myocardial infarction and their absence indicate the non-existence of myocardial infarction. Therefore there should be neither false positives, nor false negatives.

2. Size and location of body surface area showing ekg changes should be related in one way or another to size and location of the infarcted area.

3. Prediction of the histological characteristics of the infarcted region, indicating the varying stages of its development, recent, some weeks old, scarred, should be possible.

Present-day electrocardiography cannot fulfill any of these conditions. The QRS changes are non-specific. Moreover myocardial infarction patterns can be found in patients whose hearts do not show any infarction and the reverse is also true.

At a postmortem examination of 294 hearts with normal QRS in conventional leads, 38 myocardial infarctions were found (1).

It is not surprising therefore that the results of examination of large numbers of hearts with myocardial infarction demonstrate that the prediction of location and size of the infarction is often wrong.

This disturbing conclusion may indicate a fundamental shortcoming of electrocardiography.

Many years ago we tried to answer some questions about the diagnostic reliability of electrocardiography. In those days the silent zone concept was

27

'en vogue'. In dogs myocardial infarctions were made by ligation of anterior branches of the left coronary artery. On one group we studied what happened during the first 12-24 hours; in the other group the hearts were examined 6 weeks or later.

In the dogs with fresh infarction accurate location of the infarcted area was possible by epicardial exploration. In all hearts with myocardial scars, clear-cut changes in QRS were present too at its epicardial surface (2). They involved mainly the Q-wave – the duration, depth and nadir distance. The area with abnormal Q parameters accurately coincided with the infarcted area. In many instances the degree of intramural extension could be predicted from the duration of the epicardial Q-waves. A small subendocardial infarction with an area of about 1 cm² could be detected relatively easily. These experiments were performed at the anterior wall but there is no reason to expect a different conclusion for the epicardial exploration of infarction located at other sites, provided exploration occurs directly at the epicardial surface of the infarcted area. It can be expected that for infarctions located in the ventricular septum the situation is much more complex. In one revived human heart with multiple myocardial infarction, all infarctions were recognized, even one located in the posterobasal region. These results pose the problem to define those factors which greatly diminish this accurate qualitative and quantitative relationship in the intact thorax.

Our knowledge of these factors is meagre but some may be mentioned.

1. The decreased sensitivity of semidirect leads. The greater distance between precordium and anterior epicardial surface greatly decreases the details present in epicardial leads. The distance in respect to the posterior wall is even much greater.

2. Probably some regions of the heart do not influence precordial and extremity leads.

3. The pathway of normal depolarisation in the ventricles determines the type of QRS-changes in epicardial leads caused by infarction. Subendocardial or transmural infarction located in those parts of the ventricular walls, where activation of the subendocardium starts later than 30 msec, will not influence in any way the first 30 msec part of the QRS complexes recorded from other places. In the normal heart these late activated regions are situated in the posterior and basal-lateral parts of the heart and septum. Moreover the excitatory forces in these regions are moving mainly in a posterior direction, away from the commonly used precordial leads where

they are responsible for the occurrence of S. No diagnostic criteria of the S-wave for myocardial infarction are as yet known.

The pathway of ventricular excitation therefore explains why the basal-lateral part of the left ventricle may be called relatively silent because infarctions in this zone may not deform the QRS-complex with characteristic Q-wave abnormalities.

The masquerading effect of complete left bundle branch block on many clear-cut infarction patterns is generally known. But it is less wellknown that this is also true for the class of left ventricular conduction disturbances called 'hemiblock' (3). A recent inferior wall infarction pattern which was clearly visible was not present in the ekg from the same patient made about 3 weeks later, when left axis deviation was recorded. The inferior wall myocardial infarction pattern has disappeared completely. (Fig. 1 and 2).

During anterior hemiblock the excitatory forces in the anterior wall, at the very beginning of QRS, are not present. Outward moving electrical forces in the apparently intact part of the inferior ventricular wall bordering the infarcted zone, resulted in a clear-cut initial positivity in AVF.

When the fasciculus block disappeared the inferior wall pattern was again clearly visible. A posterior hemiblock would have accentuated the inferior wall pattern. If a myocardial infarction is situated in those regions of the anterior wall activated early by the anterior fascicle, a posterior hemiblock will result in decrease or disappearance of this pattern. The occurrence of anterior hemiblock will enlarge the precordial area showing Q abnormalities (Fig. 3 and 4). It has to be pointed out that the existence of conduction delay in the anterior or posterior fascicle may not increase QRS duration beyond normal limits and therefore the diagnosis of hemiblock can be missed easily in these conditions.

The excitation pattern of the left ventricle in the human heart in the first 15 msec explains these conclusions. This pattern is the result of a functional separation of the left bundle branch into 3 fascicles: the anterior, posterior and septal one (4) (Fig. 5).

In conclusion present day electrocardiography has reached the very first stages of quantification but much has to be done to improve the diagnostic reliability of the ekg, before it will be possible to predict accurately the location and size of every infarction in the human heart.

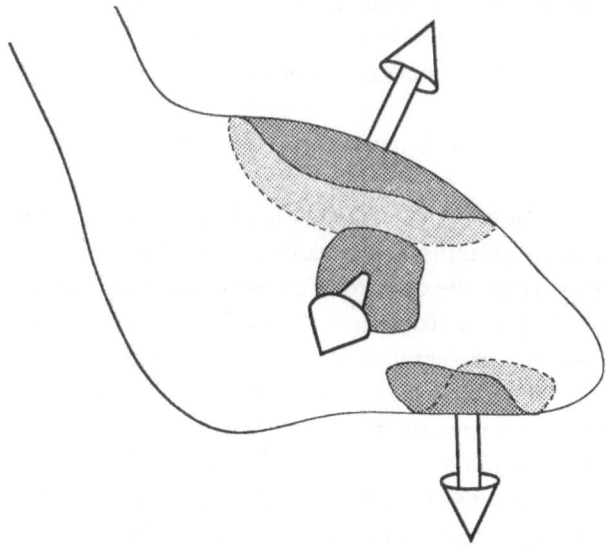

Fig. 5. Schematic representation of subendocardial areas of the left ventricle activated by the left ventricular specific conduction system during the initial 15 msec of ventricular activation. The left ventricle is depicted in the position it occupies in the thorax (anterior view).

REFERENCES

1. Horan, L. G., Flowers, N. C. & Jones, J., Significance of diagnostic Q wave of myocardial infarction. *Circulation* 43, 428 (1971).

2. Durrer, D., Van Lier, A. A. W. & Büller, J., Epicardial and intramural excitation in chronic myocardial infarction. *Amer. Heart J.* 68, 765 (1964).

3. Rosenbaum, M. B., Elizare, M. V. & Lazzari, J., *The hemiblocks*. Tampa Tracings 1970.

4. Durrer, D., Van Dam, R. Th., Freud, G. E., Janse, M. J., Meijler, F. L. & Arzbaecher, R. C., Total excitation of the isolated human heart. *Circulation* 41, 899 (1970).

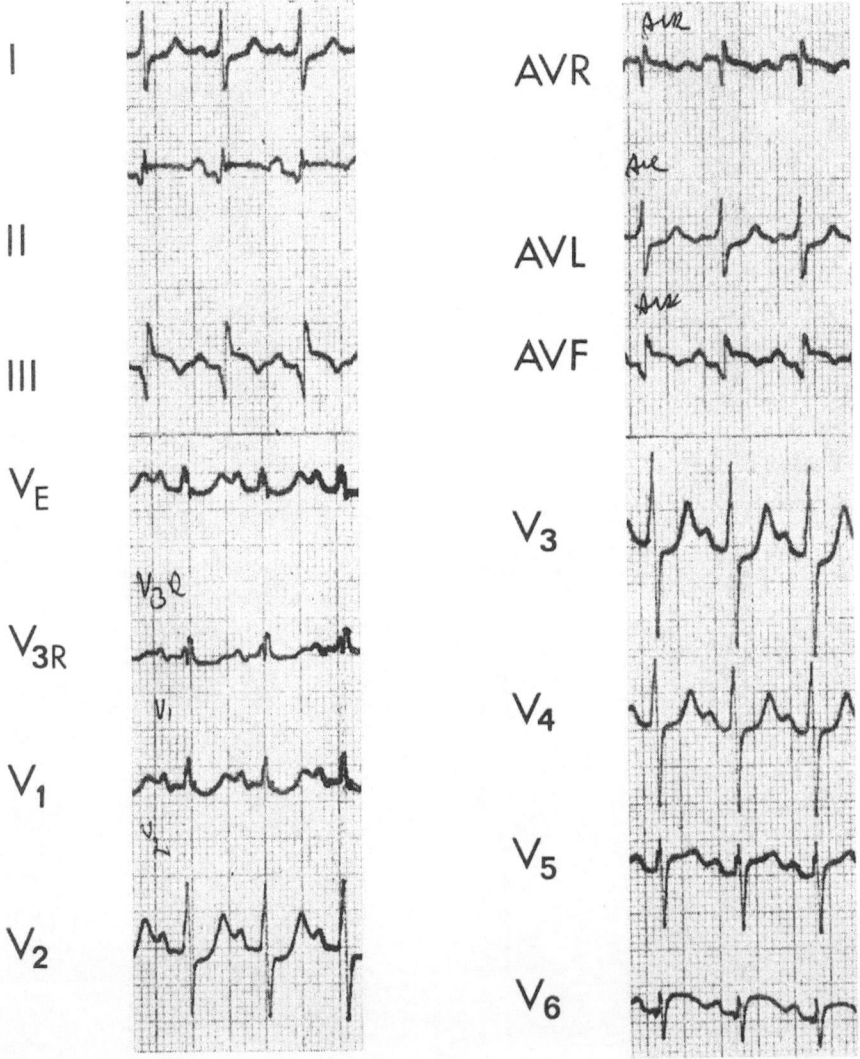

I

II

III

V_E

V_{3R}

V_1

V_2

AVR

AVL

AVF

V_3

V_4

V_5

V_6

Fig. I. Acute inferior wall infarction. QRS duration 0.08 sec.

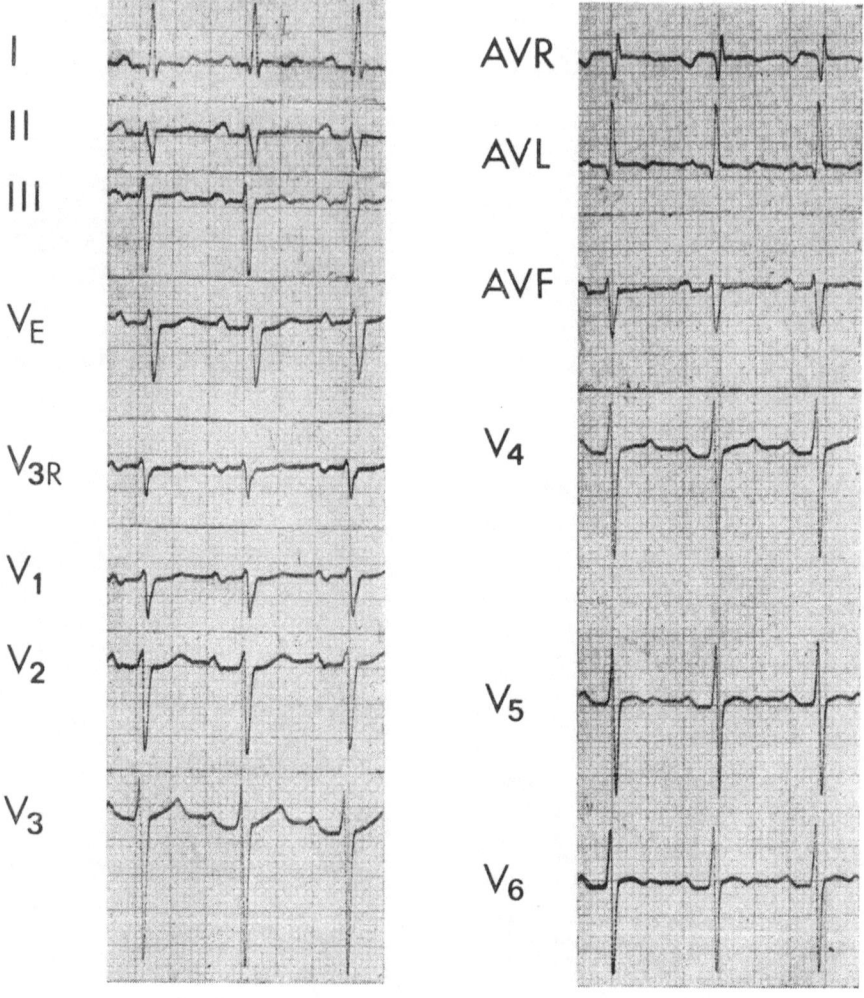

Fig. 2. Ekg from same patient as fig. 1, but left hemiblock is now present. The QRS duration is still 0.08 sec.

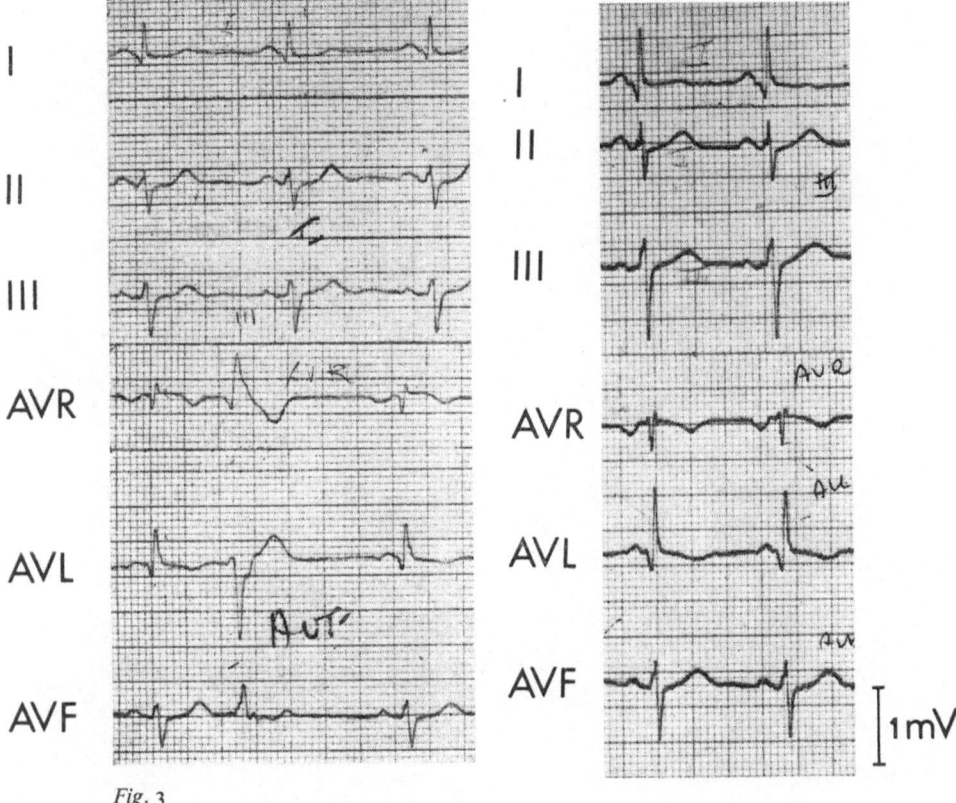

I

II

III

AVR

AVL

AVF

Fig. 3

I

II

III

AVR

AVL

AVF

1mV

Fig. 3 and 4. During normal conduction (21.4.71) a small subendocardial anterior wall infarction appears to be present. When left hemiblock occurs (19.1.71), an infarction pattern is clearly visible in a greater number of precordial leads and deepening of the Q-waves does occur.

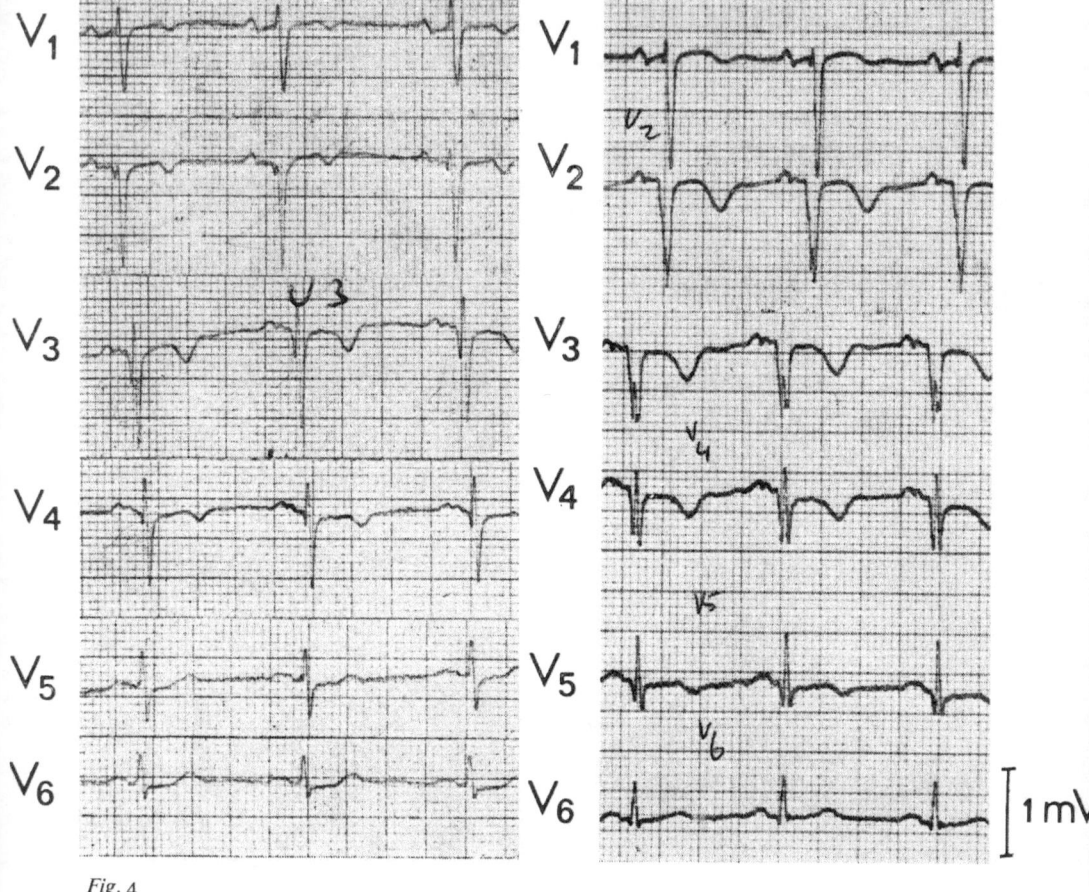

Fig. 4

QUANTITATION OF MYOCARDIAL INFARCT SIZE
AND LOCATION BY
ELECTROCARDIOGRAM AND VECTORCARDIOGRAM

R. H. SELVESTER, J. O. WAGNER AND H. B. RUBIN

SUMMARY

A method for localizing smaller infarcts into each of 12 left ventricular and septal segments is presented, along with criteria for sizing these infarcts from trival scars 1 cm in diameter to large life-threatening lesions of 8 cm in diameter. The clinical utility of being able to size infarcts with 85-90% reliability as shown here is clear cut. Lesions of 3 cm in diameter or smaller are associated with normal or near normal ventricular function and reserve. Myocardial infarcts 4-6 cm in diameter are associated with moderate ventricular disability. Lesions 7-9 cm in diameter involve 30% or more of the ventricular mass and are associated with cardiac insufficiency, pump failure, and/or low cardiac reserve.

Scars 1 and 2 cm in diameter are non-specific and can occur with inflammatory myocardial processes as well as coronary artery disease, but do not occur in the normal population. Scars 3 cm in diameter or larger are highly correlated with myocardial infarction.

INTRODUCTION

In previous work (1, 2, 3), we proposed a method for quantitating myocardial infarct size and location based on criteria developed from a computer simulation of the human heart's electrical activity. The purpose of this paper is to demonstrate the techniques of applying this tool in a daily clinical environment.

A routine method for evaluation of infarct size would be of great clinical utility in the management of patients with coronary artery disease. Homeostatic hemodynamic mechanisms are able to compensate for loss of large amounts of myocardial tissue by infarction (4). The many hemodynamic measurements studied in Myocardial Infarct Research Units establish that these compensatory mechanisms are remarkably effective until late in the course of acute progressive myocardial infarction. Few, if any, reliable measures warn of impending cardiogenic shock. Patients with cardiogenic shock are found at autopsy to have a total infarct volume in excess of 40% of the total left ventricular volume including the septum (5, 6). It, therefore, follows that a reliable electrocardiographic index of total infarct size would measure how close the patient is to the brink of impending fatal cardiogenic shock.

We have found that the criteria presented in this paper for quantitating infarct size and location now makes it possible for the clinician to predict with reasonable assurance the total infarct volume and to be aware of degrees of damage approaching that which will lead to pump failure and cardiogenic shock. In addition, the accurate determination of the location and size of a myocardial infarction makes it possible to predict with reasonable accuracy the rehabilitative prospects of the patient in the subacute phase, and permits more intelligent prescription of activity in the convalescent stage. Those patients with small infarcts in general can be ambulated sooner, require less total hospitalization and a much shorter convalescence than those with large infarcts.

PHYSIOLOGICAL BASIS

The activation fronts in the heart during ventricular depolarization generate the QRS complex of the electrocardiogram. These fronts form into complex electromotive surfaces which change over time as they propagate through the myocardium. This activation sequence in human hearts has been mapped in detail by Durrer in recent years (7). He has delineated Purkinje propagation velocity, sites of earliest activation of the ventricular myocardium and the intramyocardial propagation velocity. He has also found evidence from the intramyocardial bipolar plunge electrodes that were used for this activation sequence mapping that the dipole moment density on the active front is relatively uniform throughout the ventricle. That is, all areas contribute to the surface electrocardiogram about equally. These data combined with gross morphological anatomy of the heart provide the basis for a rational quantitative interpretation of the electrocardiogram.

This anatomical and physiological information, as well as the effects of an inhomogeneous torso (8), was incorporated into our computer simulation (3, 9, 10). This simulation now contains the major variables known to influence electric fields originating in the heart, and provides a ready method for unraveling the complex interactions of conduction abnormalities, hypertrophy of one or more chambers of the heart, and any sized infarction anywhere in the heart. For the purposes of this discussion, only normal conduction is being considered.

The total area of uncancelled front in the heart at the peak of the QRS is about 10 cm.[2] This provides the basis for relating area of front to magnitude of QRS with any lead system and hence to size of infarct when an infarct destroys a portion of the front. (3) As the infarct increases in size, it removes a greater area of activation front for a greater period of time. Size is related, then, to magnitude and duration of QRS deformity. The location of the infarct in relation to the activation fronts will determine the time in the QRS complex where this deformity will begin and the spatial direction of the deformity (2). For example, abnormal Q waves in inferior leads have for years been associated with inferior infarction and abnormal Q waves in anterior leads have been associated with anterior infarction. It now has become clear that deformities in the mid and terminal QRS complex are the result of infarction of that part of the heart activated from 30-80 msec (11, 12).

METHOD OF LOCATION AND SIZING OF INFARCT

The vector presentation allows for a more direct assessment of the time, direction, and magnitude of a QRS deformity, and the assessment of that portion of the QRS loop that is normal. The methods, however, are also applicable to the scalar ECG. For this purpose, enlarged scalars are desirable since small narrow complexes in the usual ECG record obscure small deformities in the QRS complex.

The first step in estimating the size of an infarction is to project a normal loop for comparison. If the deformity is small and of short duration, there will be a large portion of the QRS complex which is normal. This normal portion of the loop (or scalar) is then the basis for projecting an entirely normal loop for comparison. When very large areas of infarction have occurred, there will be little or none of the QRS complex that is normal. One then is required to compare the greatly deformed QRS loop to the mean normal data such as that reported by Macfarlane (13) and Draper and Pipberger (14). Here, the normal variability is carried through to the unknown as error in prediction of size and location.

In evaluating normal loops, a variant in posterior forces from 35-50 msec needs to be clarified. In our normal series, 25% have a concavity anterior in this portion of the loop. This concavity may project as much as 0.2 mV anterior to a tangential plane across the most posterior portions of the loop. This concavity shows well in both sagittal and horizontal projections. If it is smooth overall, containing no increase in high frequency notches or irregularities, and is associated with a normal T vector, then it must be considered as a normal variant. Except for this special case, VCG changes defined as 1 cm scars or larger in this paper occur in less than 2% of our 138 normals.

For the type of analysis being presented in this paper, the left ventricle is divided into its four major surfaces: 1. anterior (septal), 2. superior, 3. inferior, and 4. posterior. For the sake of convenience in locating damage into smaller subdivisions, the septum and left ventricle are further subdivided into three major regions from apex to base: apical, mesial, and basal. The following nomenclature will be used throughout and the subdivisions numbered as follows (figure 1):

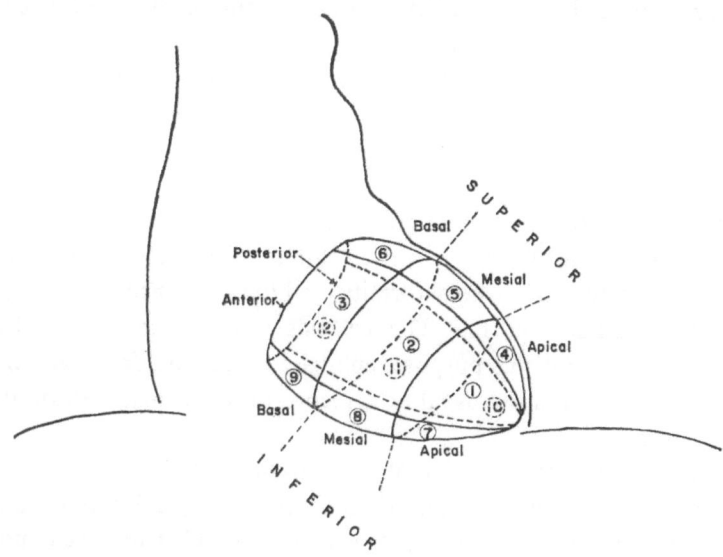

Fig. 1. Diagrammatic subdivision of the septum and left ventricle catalogued in the text.

Anterior (septal) surface
1. Antero-apical
2. Antero-mesial (Anteroseptal*)
3. Antero-basal

Superior surface
4. Supero-apical (Lateral*)
5. Supero-mesial (High lateral*)
6. Supero-basal

Inferior surface
7. Infero-apical
8. Infero-mesial (Diaphragmatic*)
9. Infero-basal (Diaphragmatic*)

Posterior surface
10. Postero-apical (True posterior*)
11. Postero-mesial (True posterior*)
12. Postero-basal

* Nomenclature in parenthesis is that used by many authors in commonly used textbooks of electrocardiography.

SIZING CRITERIA

Criteria for estimating the size of infarct incorporating both the magnitude and duration changes are presented in tables 1, 2, and 3. It is to be noted that

Table 1. vcg criteria for estimating infarct size (cube lead system).

0.1 mV deviation from a smooth loop for 10 msec = 1 cm infarct*
0.2 mV deviation from a smooth loop for 20 msec = 2 cm infarct*
0.3 mV deviation from a smooth loop for 30 msec = 3 cm infarct
0.4 mV deviation from a smooth loop for 40 msec = 4 cm infarct
0.5 mV deviation from a smooth loop for 50 msec = 5 cm infarct
0.6 mV deviation from a smooth loop for 60 msec = 6 cm infarct
0.7 mV deviation from a smooth loop for 70 msec = 7 cm infarct
0.8 mV deviation from a smooth loop for 80 msec = 8 cm infarct

* Scars 1-2 cm in diameter by these criteria are nonspecific and can occur with inflammatory myocardial processes as well as coronary artery disease, but only rarely in a normal population (2%). Scars 3 cm or larger by these criteria are highly correlated with myocardial infarction.

Table 2. vcg criteria for estimating infarct size (McFee or Frank lead systems).

0.15 mV deviation from a smooth loop for 10 msec = 1 cm infarct*
0.30 mV deviation from a smooth loop for 20 msec = 2 cm infarct*
0.45 mV deviation from a smooth loop for 30 msec = 3 cm infarct
0.60 mV deviation from a smooth loop for 40 msec = 4 cm infarct
0.75 mV deviation from a smooth loop for 50 msec = 5 cm infarct
0.90 mV deviation from a smooth loop for 60 msec = 6 cm infarct
1.05 mV deviation from a smooth loop for 70 msec = 7 cm infarct
1.20 mV deviation from a smooth loop for 80 msec = 8 cm infarct

* Scars 1-2 cm in diameter by these criteria are nonspecific and can occur with inflammatory myocardial processes as well as coronary artery disease, but occur only rarely in a normal population (2%). Scars 3 cm or larger by these criteria are highly correlated with myocardial infarction.

Table 3. ecg criteria for estimating infarct size.

Anterior infarction

Notching of R (or Q) in 1 V lead = 1 cm infarct*
Notching of R (or Q) in 2 V leads = 2 cm infarct*
Abnormal Q in 3 V leads = 3 cm infarct
Abnormal Q in 4 V leads = 4 cm infarct
Abnormal Q in 5 V leads = 5 cm infarct
Abnormal Q in 6 V leads = 6 cm infarct

Same in 6 cm with decrease in
R or absent R in V_5 but not V_6 = 7 cm infarct

Same as 7 cm with low voltage
or absent R in V_5 and V_6 = 8 cm infarct

Inferior infarction (See text)

If there is a Q of 28 msec or more in AVF, then
Frontal plane axis of 60° = 1 cm infarct*
Frontal plane axis of 40° = 2 cm infarct*

Table 3. ECG criteria for estimating size. *(continued)*

Frontal plane axis of 20°	= 3 cm infarct
Frontal plane axis of 0°	= 4 cm infarct
Frontal plane axis of −20°	= 5 cm infarct
Frontal plane axis of −40°	= 6 cm infarct
Frontal plane axis of −60°	= 7 cm infarct
Frontal plane axis of −80°	= 8 cm infarct

Posterior infarction

An R in V_1 of 40 msec or more (0.04 sec) or an rSr′ in V_1
with T axis in the horizontal of $+$ 70° to $+$ 90° with $\neq$
notching in the S wave in V_1 and in the R in V_5 and V_6

Horizontal plane axis of −20° or more	= 1-2 cm infarct*
Horizontal plane axis of −10°	= 3 cm infarct
Horizontal plane axis of $\neq$10°	= 4 cm infarct
Horizontal plane axis of $\neq$30°	= 5 cm infarct
Horizontal plane axis of $\neq$50°	= 6 cm infarct
Horizontal plane axis of $\neq$70°	= 7 cm infarct
Horizontal plane axis of $\neq$90°	= 8 cm infarct

* Scars 1-2 cm in diameter by these criteria are nonspecific and can occur with inflammatory myocardial processes as well as coronary artery disease, but occur only rarely in a
normal population (2%). Scars 3 cm or larger by these criteria are highly correlated with
myocardial infarction.

any given infarct may involve more than one segment of the aforementioned
12 subdivisions of the heart. Small scars or infarcts up to 3 cm in diameter
may be limited to one segment but lesions 4 cm in diameter or larger of
necessity involve more than one segment, and large lesions (8 cm by these
criteria) involve the equivalent of 5 total segments. The infarction may involve a portion of a number of segments, in which case the total number of
these 12 segments that may contain infarct would exceed 5 and may involve
portions of 8 or even 9 segments. In any event, these criteria do not find lesions larger than 8-9 cm which, if they are assumed to be 70-80% transmural,
will involve 40% of the total cardiac volume. This is the largest lesion compatible with life. The nomenclature for these larger lesions is maintained as
the center of the lesion.

LOCATION CRITERIA

Anterior infarction (See figures 2 and 3)

Segment 1. Antero-apical: This portion of the human heart depolarizes from
5-45 msec with fronts moving anterior, leftward and slightly inferior. Therefore, loss of these fronts will produce a deformity from the expected normal

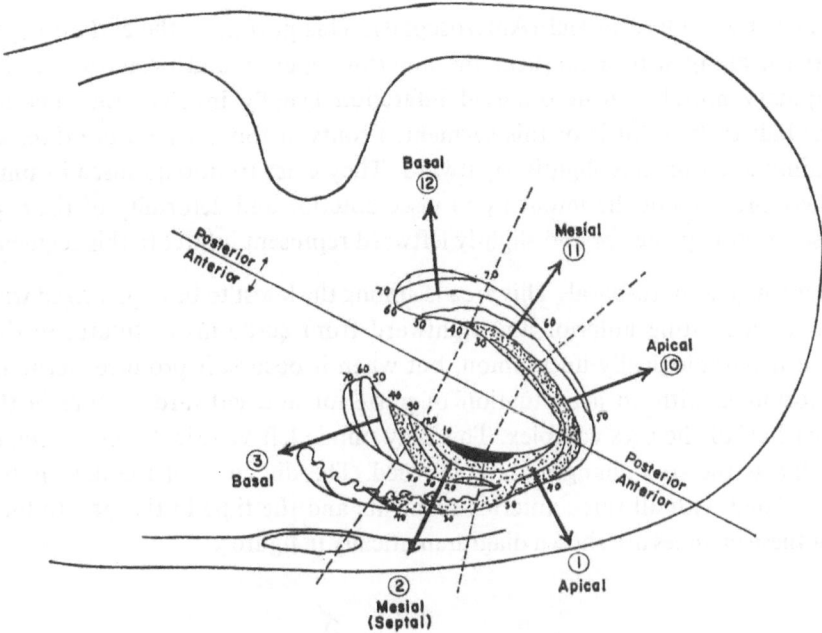

Fig. 2. Anterior wall infarction. Horizontal plane. Loop deformed posterior. If from 0-40 msec loop shows significant deformity.

1. Posterior and rightward (especially if initial 10-15 msec vectors are intact). Dx: Antero-apical infarction.
2. Posterior and leftward (especially with loss of initial 10-15 msec anterior. Dx: Anteromesial (septal) infarction.

If from 40-80 msec loop shows significant deformity.

3. Posterior and leftward (may mimic L.V.H.). Dx: Antero-basal infarct (Rare infarct pathologically).

Posterior wall infarction. Loop deformed anterior and rightward. If from 30-50 msec loop shows significant deformity.

10. Mainly rightward and slightly anterior. Dx: Postero-apical infarction.
11. Mainly anterior and slightly rightward. Dx: Postero-mesial infarction.

If from 40-80 msec loop shows significant deformity.

12. Anterior and/or rightward. Dx: Posterior-basal infarction.

that displaces the 10-40 msec portion of the loop posterior, leftward and slightly superior. When the initial 10-15 msec vectors are preserved with such deformities and the estimated size of the lesion is 3 cm in diameter or less, the area of infarction is likely limited to this segment. Examples of various sized infarcts in this location appear in our previous publications. (2, 3)

Segment 2. Antero-mesial (Anteroseptal): This portion is the earliest depolarized, along with areas near the anterior-superior and posterior-inferior papillary muscles. Antero-mesial infarction usually involves the superior one-half to two-thirds of this segment. Fronts in this segment are directed mainly anterior and slightly rightward. They exist from 0-40 msec in time. Therefore, loss of the initial 15-20 msec anterior and deformity of the 0-30 msec vectors posterior and slightly leftward represent infarct in this segment.

Segment 3. Antero-basal: This area is among the latest to be depolarized with fronts generating anterior and rightward from 40-80 msec. Infarct in this area is pathologically uncommon, but when it occurs, it produces terminal deformities with an accentuation of posterior and leftward vectors in the later half of the QRS complex. This may mimic left ventricular enlargement as far as the QRS changes are concerned. The direction of the deformities associated with all three anterior segments and the time in the QRS to look for these changes are shown diagrammatically in figure 3.

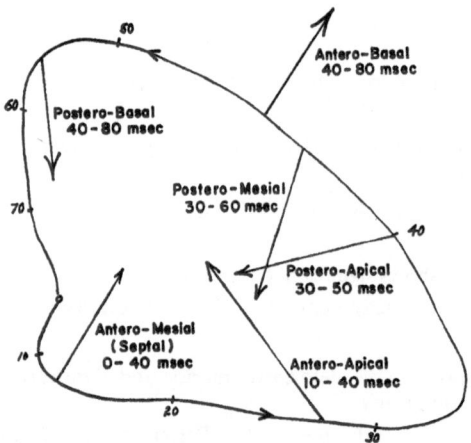

Fig. 3. Anterior-posterior infarction. Horizontal plane vcg. *Location* determined mainly by time on loop and direction of local deformity. *Size* of infarction is a function of magnitude and duration of the deformity.

Posterior infarction (See figures 2 and 3)

The posterior mesial and apical areas depolarize about simultaneously. Fronts enter both of these segments via Purkinje spread at about the same time from the three areas anteriorly, superiorly and inferiorly where the branches of the left bundle initialize ventricular activation. The fronts are directed significantly different, however, and hence the direction of the deformity from a smooth loop can be used to localize into each of these segments.

Segment 10. Postero-apical: Fronts in this segment last from 30-50 msec and are directed leftward and only slightly posterior. Infarct limited to this segment produces a deformity of the mid QRS vectors at the peak of the QRS and these deformities are directed rightward and only slightly anterior away from a normal smooth QRS loop. Examples of a number of sized lesions in this location are also published in previous papers (2, 3).

Segment 10. Postero-apical: Fronts in this segment last from 30-50 msec from 30-50 msec in this segment and infarcts that are limited mainly to this segment deform the loop mainly anterior and only slightly rightward from 30-50 msec. Posterior infarction in both apical and mesial segments produce QRS changes resembling right ventricular enlargement and at times indistinguishable from it. The common finding of increased high frequency notching and irregularities from 30-50 msec increase the probability that these changes are due to infarction. A large anterior directed symmetrical T loop when present makes infarction almost certainly the cause.

Segment 12. Postero-basal: Infarcts in this segment produce terminal 40 msec deformities in the QRS complex with displacement of terminal vectors anteriorly from their normal locations. Thus, changes resembling incomplete right bundle branch block are common. Again, the presence of high frequency notching and anterior T vectors markedly increase the probability that these changes are due to infarction.

Superior wall infarction (See figures 4 and 5)
There are simultaneous initial activation fronts in the superior wall and in the inferior wall. Those in the superior wall are larger in extent and are high at the junction of the basal one-third and the middle third. Those in the inferior wall are more towards the apex at the junction of the middle third and the lower third. Because of the location of these initial fronts, the base of the superior wall is depolarized 20 msec ahead of the base of the inferior wall and the infero-apical segment is depolarized somewhat (about 10 msec) ahead of the supero-apical segment (See figure 4).

Segment 4. Supero-apical: Since fronts in this area are directed mainly leftward and somewhat superior, from 10-50 msec QRS deformities rightward and somewhat inferior with associated high frequency irregularities from 10-50 msec are the changes diagnostic of supero-apical infarct.

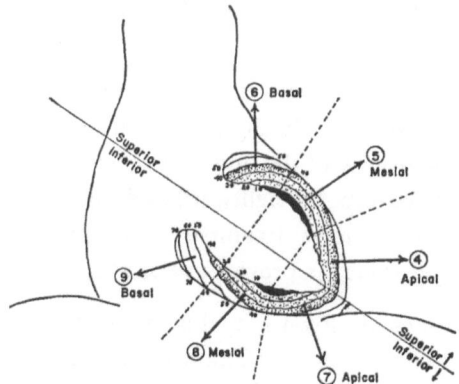

Fig. 4. Superior wall infarction. Frontal plane. Loop deformed inferior and rightward. If from 0-50 msec loop shows significant deformity.

6. Inferior and slightly leftward. Dx: Superior basal infarction (rare).

5. Inferior and rightward. Dx: Superior mesial (high lateral) infarction (common area of infarction).

4. Rightward and slightly inferior. Dx: Superior apical (lateral) infarct (common).

Inferior wall infarction. Loop deformed superior and at times leftward. If from 0-40 msec loop shows significant deformity.

7. Superior and rightward. Dx: Inferior apical infarction.

8. Superior and/or leftward. Dx: Inferior mesial infarction.

If from 40-80 msec loop shows significant deformity.

9. Superior and/or leftward (usually with left axis deviation). Dx: Inferior basal infarction.

Segment 5. Supero-mesial: Infarcts in this segment produce an initial 40 msec inferior and rightward deformity in the QRS complex. Infarction in this area is often associated with superior branch hemiblock which accentuates these initial vector changes. This will be the basis for later communications. It should be clear, however, that if the activation sequence is that of superior branch hemiblock, the size criteria will be unchanged, but timing of the location criteria will change due to the delayed activation of the superior wall. The loop of uncomplicated superior branch hemiblock should be projected for comparison.

Segment 6. Supero-basal: Infarct in this segment which is uncommon produces displacement of the initial 10-50 msec directly inferior with the usual high frequency notching in this portion of the QRS loop.

Inferior wall infarction (See figures 4 and 5)
Segment 7. Infero-apical: Infarcts here produce superior and rightward deformities with high frequency irregularities in the initial 40 msec of the QRS

loop. Isolated infarcts in this area are uncommon but infarction in this segment associated with anterior descending disease and antero-apical and/or superoapical involvement is common.

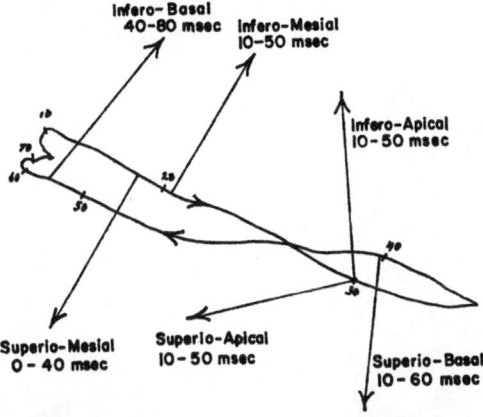

Fig. 5. Superior – Inferior infarction. Frontal plane VCG. *Location* of infarct is a function of time in the loop and the direction that the loop is deformed. *Size* of infarct is a function of the magnitude and duration of the infarct.

Segment 8. Infero-mesial: This area when infarcted produces initial 50 msec deformities superior and slightly leftward. Here, too, isolated infarction is uncommon. Association with right coronary disease and infero-basal infarct, however, is common in association with involvement of the inferior one-third of the mesial and basal septal segments.

Segment 9. Infero-basal: This is the usual area of involvement with inferior infarction and when normal conduction is present, the notching and irregularities and major deformities are in the terminal QRS vectors. From our data, it would appear that disruption of the inferior fascicles of the left bundle is common with infarction in this area, producing a variant of inferior hemiblock. In this instance, there is a smooth initial vector superior due to the unopposed early activation of the superior and anterior surfaces. Late activation fronts are directed inferior with high frequency notching through the area of infarction. This conduction abnormality associated with isolated right coronary artery disease is the basis of a more detailed report in preparation (15). Examples of various sized infero-basal infarcts with normal conduction are illustrated in figure 6. It should be noted that with normal conduction, only very large infero-basal infarcts that indeed extend to most of the inferior surface are associated with total absence of initial inferior vectors. The common association of 30-40 msec initial vectors superior and a basal infarct ventriculographically and pathologically is consistent with the hypothesis that disruption of inferior fascicles of the left bundle is common with this lesion.

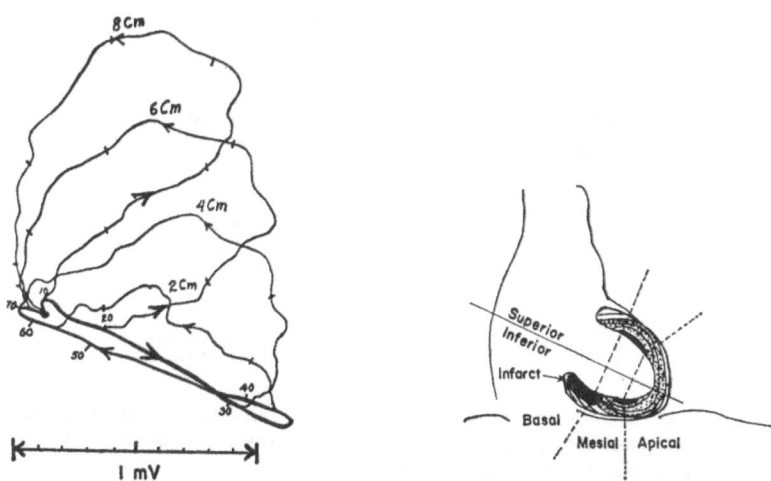

Fig. 6. Frontal plane projection of various sized infero-basal infarcts with normal conduction.

DISCUSSION

There are local proximity effects in all surface electrocardiograms. None of the VCG lead systems currently in routine use see the heart entirely as an equivalent dipole. The apex of the heart, especially segment 1 (the anteroapical segment), is geometrically close to the anterior wall of the chest and is, therefore, quite close to midprecordial scalar leads and to the anterior lead of the McFee or Frank lead system. Small antero-apical infarcts will be over-estimated as to size when these judgments are made from the McFee (or Frank) lead system by the criteria proposed in this paper. This same area is the most distant from the Cube lead system electrodes and this lead system underestimates the degree of damage by the criteria proposed for that lead system. If the size as estimated by both lead systems is averaged together, the average more closely parallels the size of the akinetic segment seen on ventriculograms.

Abildskov has argued that large infarcts occurring on opposite sides of the heart could theoretically completely neutralize each other and produce little or no change in the resultant electric field of the heart (16). Such multiple lesions, however, rarely occur anatomically in such a way as to completely neutralize each other. In data reported elsewhere (17, 18), the criteria proposed here correctly predicted the presence or absence of an akinetic segment on a ventriculogram with a 90% reliability. These criteria predicted the size and location of akinesia when present to within 1 cm with an 85% reliability. It is possible that some of the poor correlation of the 15% not accurately sized or located was due to the confounding of multiple lesions proposed by Abildskov. Another source of error is the variability in normals to which the unknown is referenced when large lesions are present.

A third source of error almost certainly is unrecognized conduction abnormalities with block in one of the major subdivisions of the left bundle branch. Such conduction abnormalities can produce major deformities in the QRS complexes. If these are unrecognized and attributed to infarction, gross errors in estimating infarct size and location would result. On the other hand, if the abnormal activation sequence is known and the surface ECG and VCG that represent this conduction abnormality are known and used for reference, then the same criteria as proposed before for sizing infarcts would still prevail.

This hypothesis was tested in a group of patients with complete left bundle branch block. A number of these patients had visible infarcts on their ventriculograms. Details of this study are being reported elsewhere, but in summary, these criteria in a small group of 20 patients with complete left bundle branch block proved as reliable in predicting the presence or absence of an akinetic segment as with normal conduction. Also, the size of the lesion and its location were predicted correctly with the same reliability.

Scars 1 and 2 cm in diameter are non-specific and can occur with inflammatory myocardial processes as well as coronary artery disease, but do not occur in the normal population. Scars 3 cm in diameter or larger are highly correlated with myocardial infarction.

REFERENCES

1. Selvester, R. H., Kalaba, R., Bellman, R., Kagiwada, H. & Collier, C. R., Simulated myocardial infarction with a mathematical model of the heart containing distance and boundary effects. In: *Proceedings Long Island Jewish Hospital. Symposium vectorcardiography*, 1965, pp. 403-410. Amsterdam 1966.

2. Selvester, R. H., Rubin, H. B., Hamlin, J. A. & Pote, W. W., New quantitative vectorcardiographic criteria for the detection of unsuspected myocardial infarction in diabetics. *Amer. Heart J.* 75, 335-348 (1968).

3. Selvester, R. H., Palmersheim, J. & Pearson, R. B., VCG inverse model for the prediction of myocardial disease. In: *Vectorcardiography* 2. Proceedings XIth International Symposium Vectorcardiography, 1970. pp. 54-65. Amsterdam 1971.

4. Swan, H. J. C., Forrester, J. S., Danzig, R. & Allen, H. N., Power failure in acute myocardial infarction. *Progr. cardiovasc. Dis.* 12, 568-600 (1970).

5. Page, D. L., Caulfield, J. B., Kastor, J. A., DeSanctis, R. W. & Sanders, C. A., Myocardial changes associated with cardiogenic shock. *New Engl. J. Med.* 285, 133-137 (1971).

6. Hanarayan, C., Bennett, M. A., Brewer, D. B. & Pentecost, B. L., Study of infarcted myocardium in cardiac shock. *Brit. Heart J.* 32, 555-556 (1970).

7. Durrer, D., van Dam, R. Th., Freud, G. E., Janse, M. J., Meijler, F. L. & Arzbaecher, R. C., Total excitation of the isolated human heart. *Circulation* 41, 899-912 (1970).

8. Selvester, R. H., Solomon, J. C. & Gillespie, T. L., Digital computer model of a total body electrocardiographic surface map; an adult male-torso simulation with lungs. *Circulation* 38, 684-690 (1968).

9. Selvester, R. H., Collier, C. R. & Pearson, R. B., Analog computer model of the vectorcardiogram. *Circulation* 31, 45-53 (1965).

10. Selvester, R. H., Kalaba, R., Collier, C. R., Bellman, R. & Kagiwada, H., A digital computer model of the vectorcardiogram with distance and boundary effects: simulated myocardial infarction. *Amer. Heart J.* 74, 792-808 (1967).

11. Young, E., Levine, H. D., Vokonas, P. S., Kemp, H. G., Williams, R. A. & Gorlin, R., The frontal plane vectorcardiogram in old inferior myocardial infarction; II. Mid-to-late QRS changes. *Circulation* 42, 1143-1162 (1970).

12. Flowers, N. C., Horan, L. G., Tolleson, W. J. & Thomas, J. R., Localization of the site of myocardial scarring in man by high-frequency components. *Circulation* 40, 927-934 (1969).

13. Macfarlane, P. W., Lorimer, A. R. & Lawrie, T. D. V., Normal ranges of modified axial lead system electrocardiogram parameters. *Brit. Heart J.* 33, 258-265 (1971).

14. Draper, H. W., Peffer, C. J., Stallmann, F. W., Littmann, D., & Pipberger, H. V., The corrected orthogonal electrocardiogram and vectorcardiogram in 510 normal men (Frank lead system). *Circulation* 30, 853-864 (1964).

15. Ciraulo, D. A., Ellis, E. J., & Selvester, R. H., *Chronic occlusive disease of the right coronary artery; a clinical angiographic*, ECG, *end* VCG *correlative study*. (In preparation).

16. Abildskov, J. A., & Klein, R. M., Cancellation of electrocardiographic effects during ventricular excitation. *Circul. Res.* 11, 247-251 (1962).

17. Selvester, R. H., Rubin, H. B., & Ellis, E. J. Vectorcardiographic and electrocardiographic estimate of myocardial damage. *Circulation* 40, Suppl. III, 182 (1969).

18. Selvester, R. H., Rubin H. B., & Wagner, J. O., Manuscript in preparation.

QUANTITATION OF THE SIZE OF
A MYOCARDIAL INFARCTION
BY DETERMINATION OF PLASMA ENZYMES

H. C. HEMKER, S. A. G. J. WITTEVEEN, W. TH. HERMENS AND
L. HOLLAAR

SUMMARY

The determination of plasma enzyme levels after a myocardial infarction proves to be a useful tool in estimating the size of an infarcted area. A quick but rough estimation can be obtained by measuring lactate dehydrogenase (LDH) (or alpha-hydroxybutyrate dehydrogenase (α-HBDH)) until the maximal value is reached about 48 hours after the infarction occurred (for patients treated with urokinase, about 30 hours). Six to eight samples taken at intervals of about six hours are sufficient for this purpose.

A more accurate estimation of the infarction size and additional information of possible clinical importance can be obtained by measuring phospho-hexose-isomerase (PHI) for about 72 hours at intervals of 3 to 4 hours and subsequent sampling once or twice a day for about 10 days.

It should be noted that treatment with urokinase enhances shed-out quite significantly. This is difficult to explain by anything other than an augmented circulation in and/or near the infarcted area.

The fate of patients suffering from myocardial infarction is determined by many factors, one of these undoubtedly being the size of the infarction.

A method for estimating the size would therefore be of considerable clinical importance. One means of such quantitation might be evaluation of the electrocardiogram. We tried to find an independent approach by studying the serum enzyme levels. At present plasma or serum enzyme levels determined after a patient is supposed to have suffered a myocardial infarction are used mainly for establishing the diagnosis. The fairly accurate enzyme determination as carried out in the clinical chemical laboratory is 'translated' in the ward as: no, small, medium or high pathological enzyme elevation. In this way much possibly useful information is lost.

In our laboratory a method was developed for assessing the extent of an infarction by evaluating plasma enzyme levels after an infarction. In principle this is an easy task; it can be compared to another pathological situation: the infusion of a coagulation factor concentrate in a hemophiliac. The rise and subsequent fall of the coagulation factor concentration in the peripheral plasma after rapid infusion can be accounted for by a two-component model in which the following processes occur:

1. Dilution in the vascular volume. The parameters determining the final concentration are:
A: amount infused
V_v: vascular fluid volume.
During this stage the coagulation factor level measured in the plasma will rise rapidly.

2. Distribution between vascular and extravascular volumes. The important parameters are:
V_e: extravascular volume
D: diffusion coefficient.

3. Disappearance of the factor from the plasma described by the breakdown constant k. This will cause the elevated protein level to resume gradually its initial value. We assumed that in the case of cardiac enzymes there is no breakdown, either thermal or chemical, of enzymes in the extravascular compartment. This assumption is based upon the fact that no appreciable breakdown of enzymes was observed during incubation of human heart tissue in physiological saline and plasma for 163 hours at 37°C.

These three processes of course occur simultaneously.

After a myocardial infarction, a similar situation occurs although it is more complicated. There is no known amount of a recognizable protein being infused practically instantaneously, but an unknown amount that appears over a certain lapse of time with a velocity which is an unknown function of time. Essentially it is this function – which we call the 'shed-out curve' – that we want to know.

Our approach is perhaps best explained in reverse order. Suppose we know the shed-out curve v(t). The total amount of enzyme(A) that is shed-out is then obtained by integrating the function:

$$A = {}_0\!\int^{\bar{t}} v(t)dt, \tag{1}$$

where we assume the shed-out to be completed at $t = \bar{t}$.

A and v(t) are expressed per unit distribution volume.

If we know the normal enzyme content of heart tissue, the size of an infarction might easily be calculated by dividing the total amount of enzyme shed-out by the normal enzyme content per gram of heart muscle.

As a first approximation, if we neglect diffusion to the extravascular compartment, the situation can be described by the following formula:

$$\frac{dC_v(t)}{dt} = v(t) - k.C_v(t), \tag{2}$$

where $C_v(t)$ = concentration of enzyme in the vascular compartment and

$$\frac{dC_v(t)}{dt} = \text{change in } C_v(t) \text{ per unit time.}$$

When shed-out is completed, this formula reduces to:

$$\frac{dC_v(t)}{dt} = - k.C_v(t), \tag{3}$$

whereby the concentration $C_v(t)$ decreases exponentially.

Thus by plotting the measured enzyme levels as a semi-logarithmic curve, starting at that point where one can be sure shed-out has stopped (app. 30 hours after the infarction occurred), the breakdown coefficient k can be determined. From the $C_v(t)$ curve one can also obtain

$$\frac{dC_v(t)}{dt}$$

and knowing k, the shed-out curve is determined by formula (2).

In reality one cannot neglect the extravascular compartment, which makes things considerably more complicated. Now the following set of equations must be substituted for formula 2:

$$\frac{dC_v(t)}{dt} = v(t) - k.C_v(t) + \frac{D}{V_v} (C_e(t) - C_v(t)) \text{ and} \tag{4a}$$

$$\frac{dC_e(t)}{dt} = \frac{D}{V_e} (C_v(t) - C_e(t)), \tag{4b}$$

where D is the diffusion constant determining the enzyme exchange between the two compartments. $C_e(t)$ = concentration of enzyme in the extravascular compartment.

The change in concentrations by diffusion has been included in equation (4). As mentioned above, there is no enzyme breakdown in the extravascular compartment which means that the change in concentration in the extravascular compartment due to diffusion is given by equation (4b) only.

Many authors assume two diffusion constants, one determining the enzyme transport from the vascular to the extravascular compartment and one for the reverse transport. This is motivated by rather vague terms like 'irreversibly transported enzymes' or 'actively transported enzymes'.

In our opinion this is not only physically unrealistic, it is also a serious obstacle because the extra parameter introduced makes practically impossible the already difficult task of extricating the unknown parameters from the measured curves.

In order to find the shed-out curve $v(t)$, equation (4a) has to be solved, which implies that $C_e(t)$ has to be known. Therefore one must solve (4b) first.

A few calculations now show that after shed-out has stopped, the decrease in $C_v(t)$ is a double exponential function of time; in other words the semi-logarithmic plot yields two slopes K_1 and K_2, having a difference in magnitude:

$$K_1 - K_2 = 2 \sqrt{\tfrac{1}{4}\left(k + \frac{D}{V_e} + \frac{D}{V_v}\right)^2 - \frac{Dk}{V_e}}. \tag{5}$$

By determining this difference for several patients (differing in vascular fluid volume V_v), one can in principle calculate the unknown parameters V_e, D and k. In order to make this feasible, $K_1 - K_2$ must satisfy several requirements.

First, the values of D, V_e and k must be such that $K_1 - K_2$ is not too small to measure. For several enzymes this unfortunately proved to be the case.

If on the other hand the value of either K_1 or K_2 is too high, the rapid part of the decrease will be completed too soon after shed-out stops to be measurable. This is so especially because shed-out diminishes gradually; it does not stop suddenly. To circumvent this complication, we tried a rapid infusion of 250 ml plasma with elevated enzyme levels (taken from the same patient about 24 hours after infarction, when the enzyme level is close to its peak).

The infusion was given one month after the infarction, when the enzyme level had resumed its normal value, and subsequent plasma samples were taken to measure enzyme disappearance. This approach was not continued, however, because the rise in enzyme level was too small for accurate determination of the disappearance of the enzymes.

RESULTS

For 13 patients the enzyme levels were determined for the following enzymes:

Glutamic-oxaloacetic transaminase EC 2.6.1.1. (GOT), lactate dehydrogenase EC 1.1.1.27 (LDH), alfa-hydroxybutyrate dehydrogenase EC 1.1.1.30 (α-HBDH), phospho-hexose-isomerase EC 5-3-1-9 (PHI) and creatine phosphokinase EC 2.7.3.2. (CPK).

The considerable amount of data acquired were analysed using an IBM 1800-computer. Of these patients only 7 provided useful material; the remainder showed major irregularities in the enzyme level curves due to reinfarction, liver abnormalities, fever, etc.

Of these 5 enzymes, only PHI shows a clear-cut biphasic decrease, resulting in the following values for D, V_e and k:

$D_{PHI} = 0.012 \pm 0.007 \, l/h$

$V_e = (0.25 \pm 0.03) \, V_v \, 1$

k ranges from $k = 0.11 \pm 0.01$ to $k = 0.026 \pm 0.005$

The shed-out curves in figure 1 show the very interesting fact that patients treated with urokinase have a much more rapid shed-out than patients not treated in this way. The urokinase was given by injection (500.000 U in 10 minutes) and continuous infusion (18 hours of 250.000 U per hour).

This fact might be of clinical importance because the increased flow of blood through the infarcted area, which can be held responsible for the quicker removal of material from the damaged cells, will also provide a larger supply of oxygen and nutrients for this same area.

As explained above, the normal enzyme content of heart muscle must be known in order to quantify the infarction. This was determined using pieces of fresh heart muscle obtained during surgery.

As a result we found infarction sizes ranging from 11 to 35 grams of destroyed heart tissue. The estimated accuracy of these weights is about 5%.

DISCUSSION

The first point of discussion is the rather low value for the extravascular volume of about 25% of the vascular volume. Recent data (1, 2) on the distribution space of radioactively labelled prothrombin (M = 68.000) and

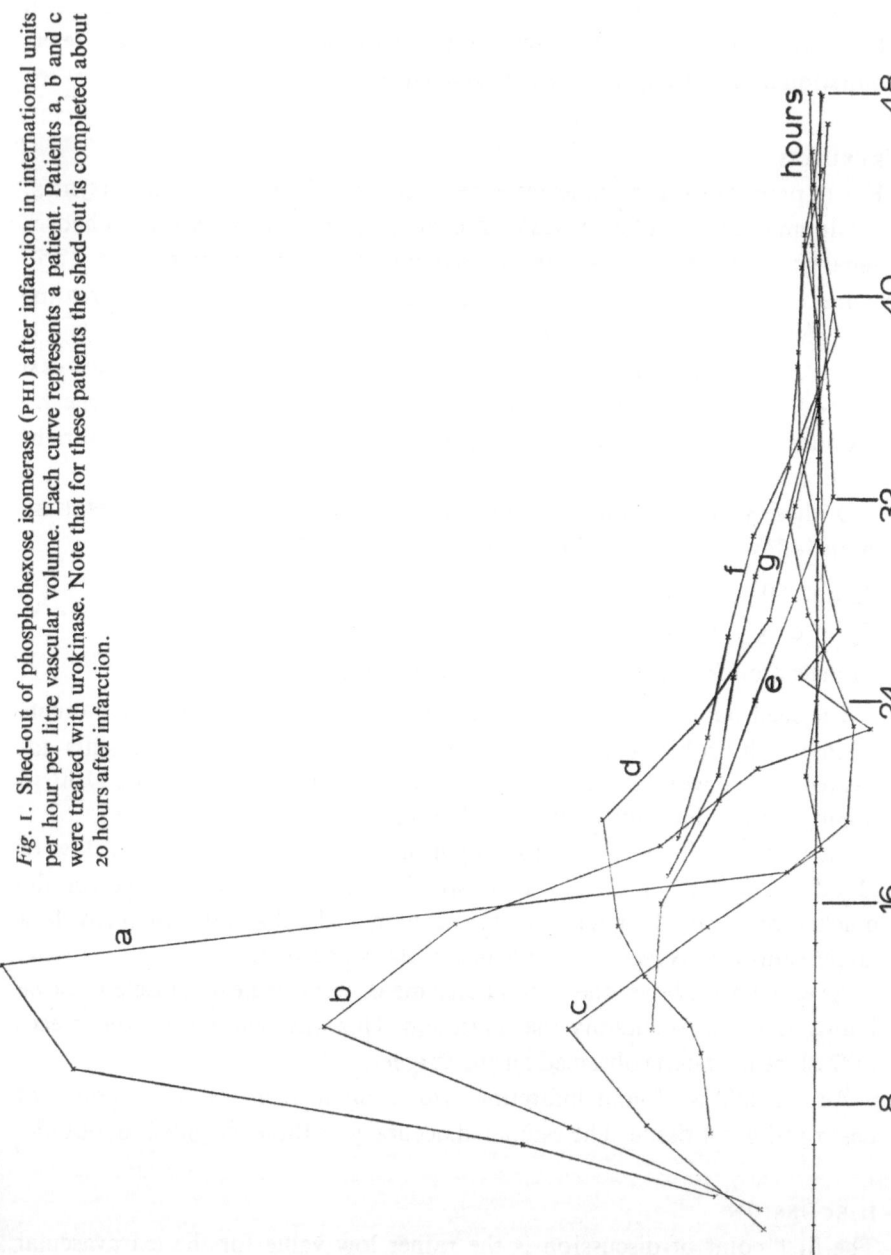

Fig. 1. Shed-out of phosphohexose isomerase (PHI) after infarction in international units per hour per litre vascular volume. Each curve represents a patient. Patients a, b and c were treated with urokinase. Note that for these patients the shed-out is completed about 20 hours after infarction.

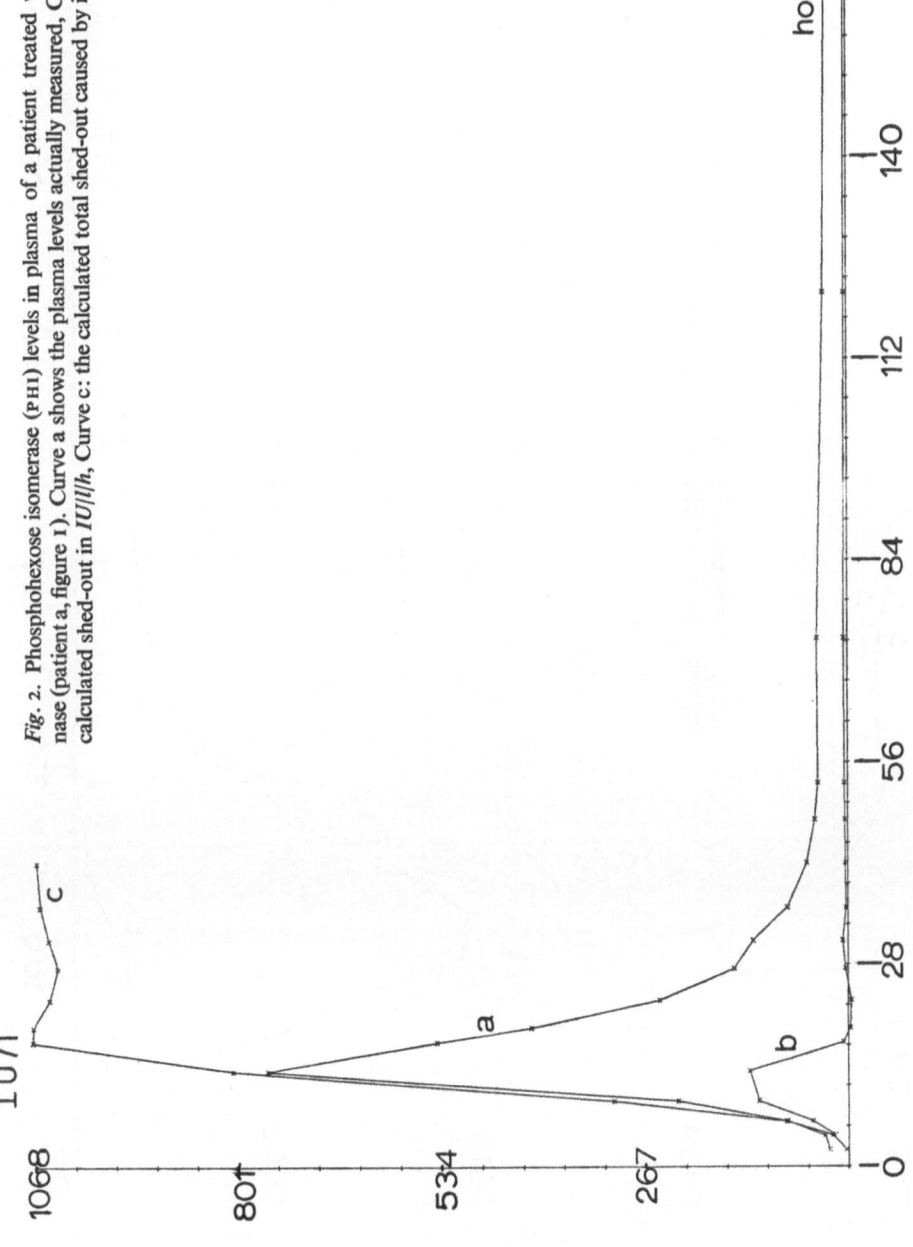

Fig. 2.. Phosphohexose isomerase (PHI) levels in plasma of a patient treated with uroki-nase (patient a, figure 1). Curve a shows the plasma levels actually measured, Curve b: the calculated shed-out in *IU/l/h*, Curve c: the calculated total shed-out caused by infarction

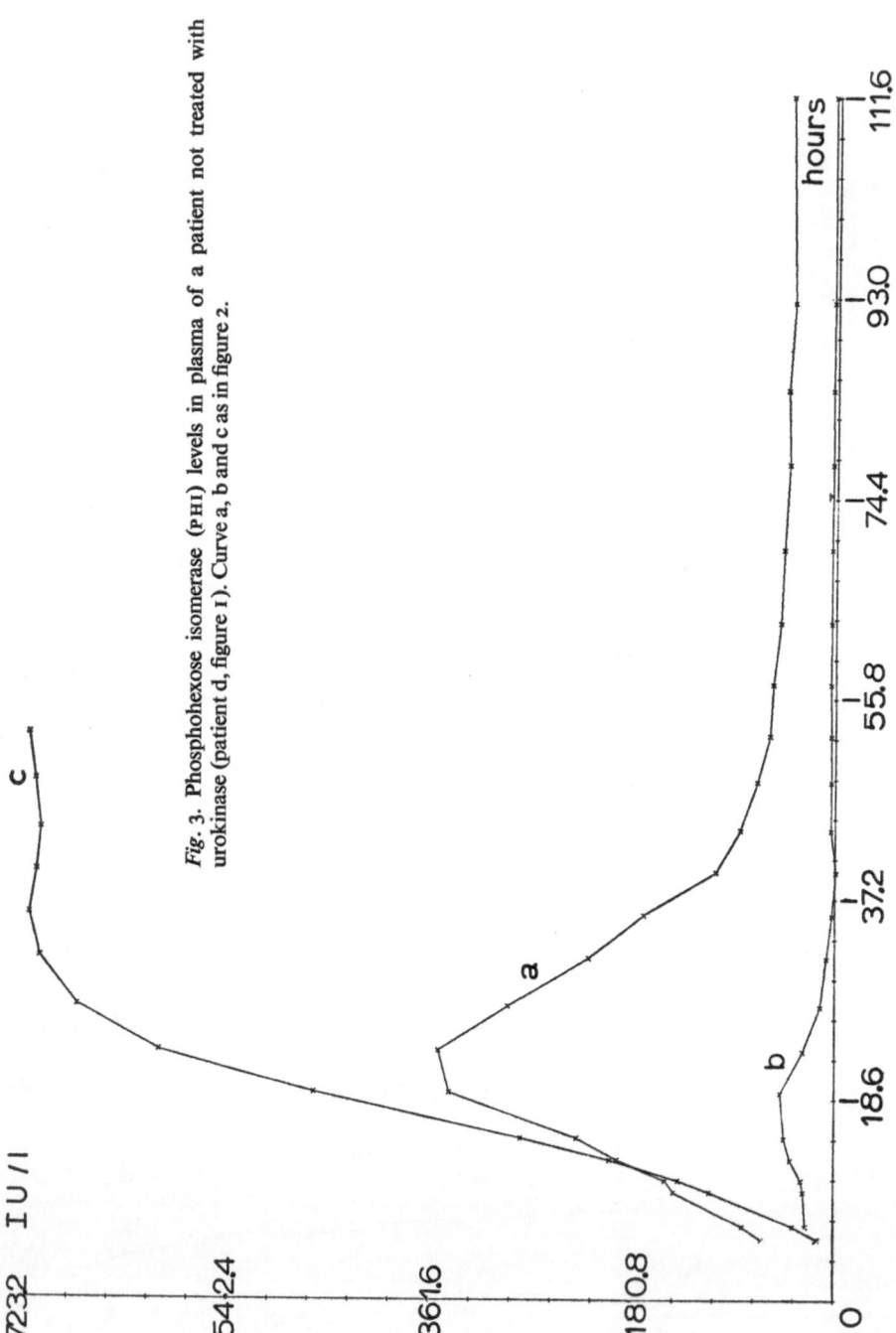

Fig. 3. Phosphohexose isomerase (PHI) levels in plasma of a patient not treated with urokinase (patient d, figure 1). Curve a, b and c as in figure 2.

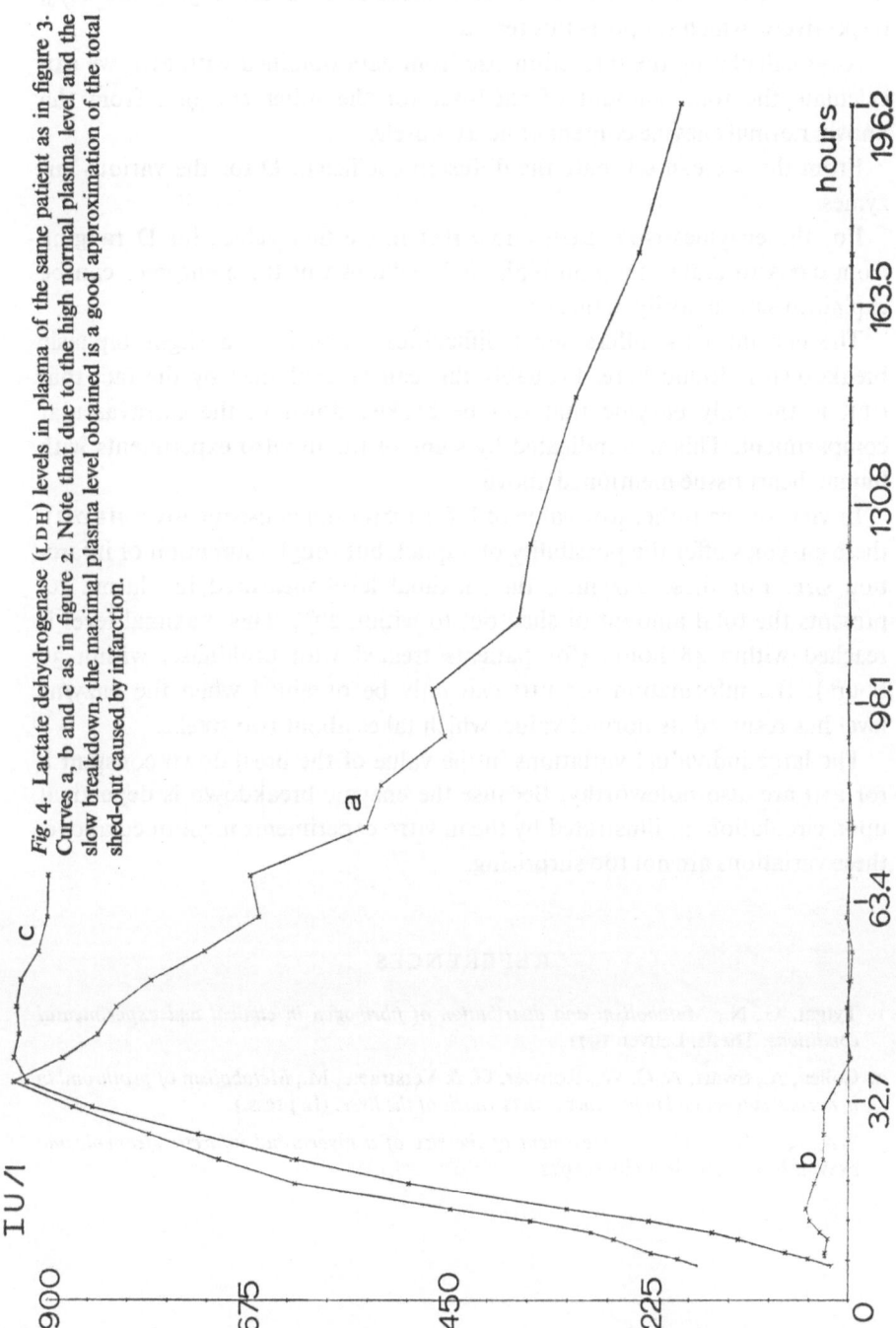

Fig. 4. Lactate dehydrogenase (LDH) levels in plasma of the same patient as in figure 3. Curves a, b and c as in figure 2. Note that due to the high normal plasma level and the slow breakdown, the maximal plasma level obtained is a good approximation of the total shed-out caused by infarction.

fibrinogen (M = 314.000) yielded extravascular volumes of 50% and 28%, respectively, which supports this result.

After calculating the infarction size from data obtained with PHI, we can calculate the total amount of shed-out for the other enzymes from the known normal enzyme content of heart muscle.

From this we can estimate the diffusion coefficient D for the various enzymes.

For the enzymes GOT, LDH and α-HBDH, we find values for D ranging from 0.005 to 0.015; the non-biphasic breakdown of these enzymes can be explained satisfactorily in this way.

The enzyme CPK offers some difficulties. Sometimes a slight biphasic breakdown is found here. Probably this can be explained by the fact that CPK is the only enzyme that can be broken down in the extravascular compartment. This was indicated by some of the in vitro experiments with human heart tissue mentioned above.

In view of the rather low value of k for LDH (and consequently α-HBDH), these enzymes offer the possibility of a quick but rough estimation of infarction size. For these enzymes, the maximal level measured in plasma represents the total amount of shed-out to within 20%. This maximal level is reached within 48 hours (for patients treated with urokinase, within 30 hours); the information for PHI can only be obtained when the enzyme level has resumed its normal value, which takes about two weeks.

The large individual variations in the value of the breakdown constant k for PHI are also noteworthy. Because the enzyme breakdown is dependent upon circulation, as illustrated by the in vitro experiments mentioned above, these variations are not too surprising.

REFERENCES

1. Tytgat, G. N., *Metabolism and distribution of fibrinogen in clinical and experimental conditions.* Thesis. Leuven 1971.

2. Collen, A., Swart, A. C. W., Rouvier, G. & Verstraete, M., *Metabolism of prothrombin in normal subject and in patients with cirrhosis of the liver.* (In press.)

3. Witteveen, S. A. G. J., *Assessment of the size of a myocardial infarction from plasma enzyme levels.* Thesis, Leiden 1972

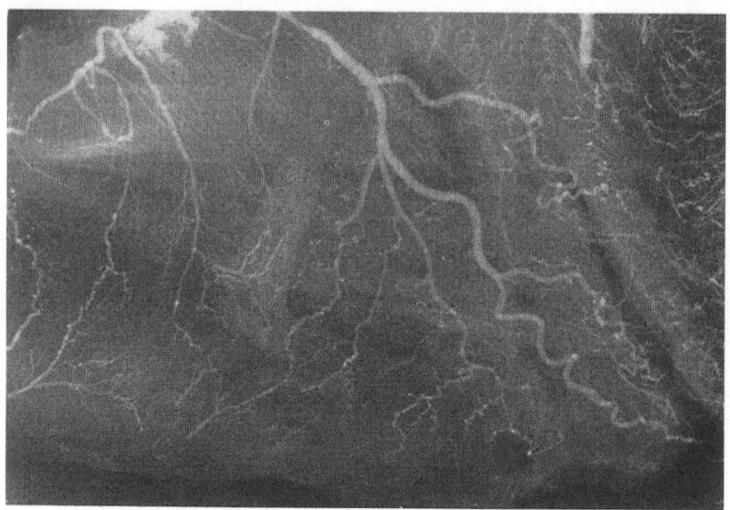

Fig. 1. Collateral vessels in a human heart with chronic coronary artery occlusion. Sub-branches of the right coronary artery are connected with the peripheral end of the occluded left anterior descending branch (not shown) via epicardial and endocardial collaterals. Note the 'corkscrew' tortuosity of these vessels.

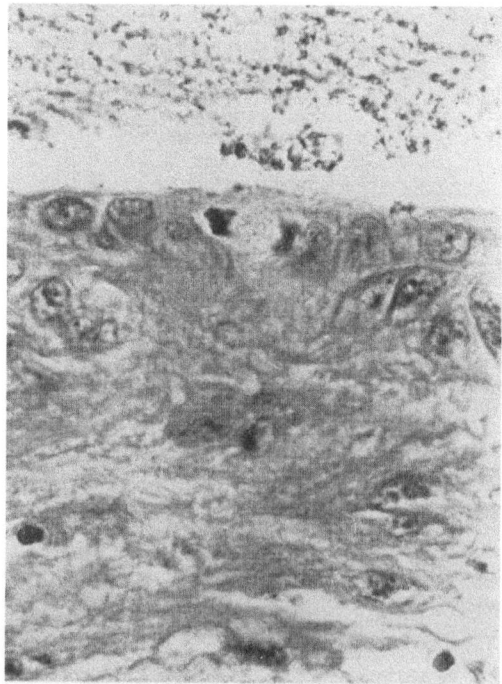

Fig. 2. Mitosis of a subintimal smooth muscle cell in a collateral vessel from a dog's heart with chronic coronary artery occlusion.

COLLATERAL CIRCULATION

W. SCHAPER

Coronary artery occlusion does not always lead to myocardial infarction. A classical example was published by Blumgart et al. in 1940 (1) of a 52-year-old man who died from a cerebral hemorrhage. Injection of the coronary arteries with a radio-opaque medium showed four occluded and four severely stenosed coronary arterial branches, but no trace of a myocardial infarct.

Collaterals and anastomoses had prevented the infarct. Many such cases have been described in the literature especially by Molnar et al. (2), Ravin and Geever (3) and by Baroldi (4). I have also encountered a few cases during my studies in human cardiac pathology. The first case is a 55-year-old man who died of silicosis. The postmortem arteriogram showed an old re-canalized obstruction of the left anterior descending artery. Two large epicardial collaterals interconnected subbranches of the LAD with those of the left circumflex artery. There was only slight scarring in the interventricular septum but no clear-cut infarct. The patient had never suffered from angina.

Another case is a 60-year-old male who died of stomach cancer. The left anterior descending coronary artery was completely obstructed but 2 large collaterals by-passed the obstacle and a myocardial infarct could not be detected.

It is at present not known in how many cases collaterals prevent myocardial infarcts or reduce their size. It is also not clearly understood which factors govern the enlargement of collaterals.

My own studies have led to some conclusions which I will try to support by experimental evidence.

1. The degree and rate of enlargement of collaterals and anastomoses depend on the size of the genetically determined pre-existent network of anastomoses. This network is located at the epicardial surface of the dog's heart and the endocardial surface of pig and human hearts. Dogs usually have numerous collaterals; these vessels are easily demonstrated in the

human heart although to a somewhat lesser extent; they are poorly developed in the pig heart. Sheep do not have collaterals or anastomoses.

2. The enlargement of the small precapillary anastomoses into relatively large collateral arteries is time-dependent and varies from species to species. Rapidly occurring coronary artery occlusion leads invariably and in all species to myocardial infarction. Whenever the progress of coronary arterial narrowing is slow, the enlargement of collaterals can follow and death and infarction can be avoided. When the rate of narrowing is sufficiently slow, infarction can be avoided altogether in the event of a large coronary artery occlusion. The time constant of this process varies from species to species. When a large coronary artery narrows progressively and occlusion does not occur prior to the 4th week after onset of narrowing, chances are that a canine heart will not develop a myocardial infarct. In the porcine and human heart, this may easily take 3-4 months but these are mere impressions which cannot at present be based on facts.

3. We have shown that the enlargement of collaterals and anastomoses is not due to passive stretch but rather to active growth. This was proven by the observation of smooth muscle mitosis and by the demonstration of DNA-synthesis in the vascular smooth muscle of growing arteries. We could show that the highest rate of smooth muscle division is about once every 24 hours in the case of reversible muscular ischemia.

In summary this means that a myocardial infarction can be avoided:

a. when the rate of coronary arterial narrowing is sufficiently slow;
b. when the pre-existent network of collaterals is sufficiently large;
c. when the rate of cell division in the vascular wall is sufficiently fast and;
d. when at least one artery remains sufficiently normal to function as a donor artery for collaterals.

It becomes clear that the concerted action of all factors is difficult to achieve which is one of the reasons for the present high morbidity in myocardial infarction.

Since this course deals with quantification, I shall try to give some quantitative information with regard to the function of collaterals.

Three aspects of the collateral circulation can be expressed quantitatively.

1. The transmission of the perfusion pressure over the lumped collateral vessels.
2. The coronary collateral flow and
3. The dilatory reserve of the collateral-dependent resistance vessels.

The pressure transmission over collaterals is poor immediately after abrupt ligation of a coronary artery. This so-called peripheral coronary pressure(PCP) drops to values of about 10% of the perfusion pressure after arterial ligation.

This pressure drop is much less pronounced when arterial narrowing occurs slowly, i.e. within a period of weeks or months. In this case a clear-cut dip in the PCP is not recognized, instead it decreases gradually to about 80% of the diastolic perfusion pressure. This means that a pressure gradient ratio of about 20% persists even after years of chronic coronary artery occlusion.

It is our experience that the height of the diastolic PCP correlates well with the average diameter and number of collaterals and anastomoses.

The coronary collateral flow can be measured in animals with chronic coronary artery occlusion at various time intervals after slowly occurring occlusion. We used the Radio-Xenon and the Radio-Krypton method in either the acute open-chested or the chronic preparation with chronic in-dwelling coronary artery catheters. Collateral flow is very low immediately after an abrupt ligation, i.e. about 10% of normal coronary flow in dogs and about 1% of the required flow in pigs. In slowly occurring coronary artery occlusion the collateral flow shows only a transient decrease and then returns rapidly to normal values.

When the rate of arterial narrowing is slow, i.e. several months, there is never a measurable reduction in collateral flow. Most of our own studies were conducted in animals where the largest coronary artery occluded over a period of about 3 weeks. In these animals a slight reduction in collateral-dependent perfusion was noted which lasted only several days; this was tolerated without myocardial infarction. This means: normal myocardial perfusion is restored faster than the peripheral coronary pressure.

The dilatory capacity of the collateral-dependent resistance vessels is, however, severely reduced in the early period after coronary artery occlusion.

We tested the dilatory capacity of the collateral-dependent resistance vessels by studying the distribution of radioactively labelled Tracer-Microspheres after drug-induced coronary vasodilation.

Tracer- Microspheres are plastic beads of precapillary size (i.e. 15 micron) which have a specific gravity similar to that of blood. They travel, when injected into the left atrium, with the bloodstream and are trapped in the precapillary arterioles. The organ-radioactivity is proportional to the quantity of trapped spheres which in turn is proportional to that fraction of the cardiac output which went to the organ under study. At present 5 differently labelled microspheres are available.

Our working hypothesis with regard to the dilatory capacity of the collateral-dependent resistance vessels is as follows: when the occluded coronary artery is functionally and completely replaced by collaterals, any type of induced general coronary vasodilation must result in a completely homogeneous distribution of myocardial flow. When the occluded coronary artery is not completely and functionally replaced by collaterals, i.e. when relatively large pressure gradients persist, the induced vasodilation is expected to produce a non-homogeneous myocardial flow to the disadvantage of the collateral-dependent area. This is called, for reasons of analogy, a Myocardial Steal Syndrome (MSS). MSS could be produced in animals with chronic large coronary artery occlusion where collaterals had effectively prevented an infarct but where the dilatory reserve was still somewhat compromised.

The mechanism of MSS is difficult to understand. I tend to believe that the increase in flow causes a pressure drop over that artery which also functions as a donor artery for collaterals. In this way, the pressure head for the collaterals is severely reduced which may cause a non-homogeneous distribution of myocardial flow.

REFERENCES

1. Blumgart, H. L., Schlesinger, M. J. & Davis, D., Studies on the relation of the clinical manifestations of angina pectoris, coronary thrombosis and myocardial infarction to the pathologic findings, with particular reference to the significance of collateral circulation. *Amer. Heart J.* 19, 1 (1940).

2. Molnar, W., Meekstroth, C. V., Nelson, S. W. & Booth, R. W., Transcarotid coronary arteriography in man with emphasis on intercoronary arterial anastomoses. *Radiology* 75, 185 (1960).

3. Ravin, A. & Geever, E. F., Coronary arteriosclerosis, coronary anastomoses and myocardial infarction. *Arch. intern. Med.* 78, 125 (1946).

4. Baroldi, G. Mantero, O. & Scomazzoni, G., The collaterals of the coronary arteries in normal and pathologic hearts. *Circulat. Res.* 4, 223 (1956).

DISCUSSION

Snellen: Dr. Schaper presented various aspects of collateral circulation and their effects on coronary circulation as a whole. At the same time he reminded us that we must not rely too heavily on the coronary angiogram when assessing the extent of the infarcted area. I would ask Dr. Durrer to discuss the differences of opinion between Dr. Selvester and himself.

Durrer: I think this disagreement is not so very pronounced. First of all we must realize that Dr. Selvester formulated the same conclusions as I did, namely that our knowledge of electrocardiographic changes in myocardial infarction in routinely used leads is insufficient. We can point out the exact location of the regions which do not provide any information at all about the existence of myocardial function. Secondly, the assertion that a hemiblock as well as an anterior hemiblock or posterior block adversely influences the diagnostic accuracy of the ECG will be readily accepted by Dr. Selvester, I think. The point of difference concerns the influence of slight changes in conduction in the anterior and posterior fascicle on the myocardial infarction pattern. We shall investigate this in the near future.

Snellen: It is obvious that there is also room for the biochemical estimation.

Durrer: I think the work of Dr. Hemker is of very great importance and offers a very good estimate of the size of the infarcted area. The figures shown agree closely with the amount of tissue ordinarily involved in myocardial infarction. But what I want to ask you is this. Sometimes myocardial infarction is not instantaneous, but several consecutive 'incidents' occur before the occlusion is complete. Have you ever seen an indication of this type of development of myocardial infarction?

Hemker: What we measure is the result of necrosis. So until there is necrosis, we see nothing. But we have several cases in which the shed-out curve did not consist of one phase but was biphasic or triphasic. This is illustrated in the graph you see here.

We must assume that in this case necrosis occurred in 2 phases. I did not

touch upon this subject because the details still have to be worked out, but
actually you learn quite a lot from closer observation of the shed-out curves.

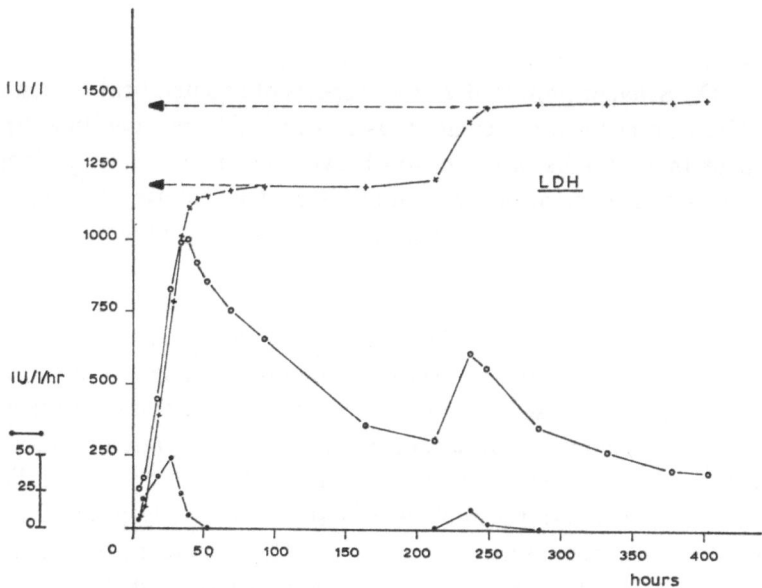

Biphasic shed-out of LDH in a case of early re-infarction.

Selvester: What I would like to dangle in front of Dr. Durrer's nose and
mine for the next few years is that if we can quantify the electrical signal
(and it looks like we now have the tools in hand), we will be able to determine the damage to the myocardium quantitatively. Then with the enzyme
shed-out curves we might be able to predict how much of that damage is old
and how much of it is recent. To do away with the notion that we ought to
treat all people alike is the real plea I would like to make to the clinicians
here. Perhaps we can differentiate treatment on the basis of assessments of
infarction size. Many patients with small infarcts can be actively rehabili-
tated in about 6 weeks. So far we have handled about 100 cases in this way,
without significant problems of arrhythmia or extension of infarction.

CHAPTER 2

EXERCISE TESTS

ELECTROCARDIOGRAPHY DURING EXERCISE IN PATIENTS WITH CORONARY SCLEROSIS AND NORMAL ELECTROCARDIOGRAM AT REST. COMPARISON WITH FINDINGS FROM CORONARY ARTERIOGRAPHY

C. A. ASCOOP AND M. L. SIMOONS

It is a well-known fact that patients with anginal complaints often show a normal electrocardiogram taken at rest, although they may have severe coronary sclerosis as disclosed by anatomopathologic examinations or coronary arteriography. In such patients with normal resting electrocardiograms, we were interested in the additional diagnostic information from the electrocardiogram during the exercise test.

Out of about 1000 patients subjected to coronary arteriography (CAG) because of anginal complaints, we were able to select 96 patients with a normal electrocardiogram taken at rest.

On all these patients, a graded exercise test (GXT) was performed and on 91 of them, a Master step test. The Master step test was slightly modified in that only one lead (CB5) was recorded. The GXT was performed on a bicycle ergometer and the external load was increased 10 watts every minute until one of the criteria to stop appeared. Throughout the exercise phase and the recovery phase, a 12-lead electrocardiogram was continuously recorded. An exercise test was deemed positive if a junction depression of ≥ 0.1 mV with respect to the preceeding PR line was provoked by the exercise, and if the ST segment sloped downwards or was horizontal over at least an 80 msec interval.

The purpose of this study was to compare these two exercise tests and to assess their additional diagnostic value in patients with a normal electrocardiogram taken at rest. The results of these exercise tests were gauged against the objective standard of reference provided by the CAG*. The angiogram was judged to be positive if a narrowing of over 50% was found in any

* All patients underwent selective coronary arteriography following Sones' technique, using multiple left and right anterior oblique projections.

of the main coronary vessels. Prediction and truth were confronted in contingency tables (1).

Table 1. Relation between coronary arteriogram (CAG) and two-step test
Fraction correct-positive = 0.33
Fraction correct-negative = 0.93
Index of merit = 0.26 ($\pm$ 0.10)

CAG \ Two-step test	+	−	
+	13	26	(39)
−	4	48	(52)
	(17)	(74)	(91)

Table 1 demonstrates the diagnostic performance of the two-step test in which there were 13 correct-positive, 48 correct-negative, 26 false-negative and 4 false-positive predictions. The fraction correct-positive = 0.33 (sensibility of the test) and the fraction correct-negative = 0.93 (specificity of the test) yield an Index of merit of 0.93 + 0.33 — 1 = 0.26.

Table 2 represents the diagnostic performance of the GXT which scored 26 correct-positive, 49 correct-negative, 18 false-negative and 3 false-positive predictions. The results are compared in table 3. It appears that the GXT is distinctly superior to the two-step test because of the higher fraction of correct-positive cases. One might suppose that in our material the GXT compared favourably to the two-step test because more leads were employed. It seems unlikely however that this could be the only explanation since in 86% of the cases rated as positive by the GXT, an ischemic response was found in lead V5: if only this lead were recorded, the GXT would still score definitely higher than the two-step test.

In table 4, it can be seen that our results are well in agreement with the findings reported by other investigators applying the same type of graded exercise test and similar criteria. It is of interest that the authors who had the highest sensibility in their exercise test also had the lowest specificity. From table 4, it also appears that in our series the diagnostic performance, in-

Table 2. Relation between coronary arteriogram (CAG) and graded exercise test (GXT).

Fraction correct-positive : $\dfrac{26}{44} = 0.59$

Fraction correct-negative: $\dfrac{49}{52} = 0.94$

Index of merit: $\dfrac{26}{44} + \dfrac{49}{52} - 1 = 0.53 \ (\pm 0.08)$

GXT / GAC	+	−	
+	26	18	(44)
−	3	49	(52)
	29	(67)	(96)

Table 3. Comparative results and predicting value of two-step test and graded exercise test (bicycle test).

	Correct-positive fraction	Correct-negative fraction	Index of merit (T)
Two-step test	0.33	0.93	0.26 ($\pm$ 0.10)
Bicycle test	0.59	0.94	0.53 ($\pm$ 0.08)

Table 4. Results of graded exercise test and comparison with coronary arteriographic findings by different authors.

	Number of patients	Fraction correct- positive	negative	Index of merit (T)
Kassebaum, Sutherland and Judkins (3)	68	0.51	0.96	0.47 ($\pm$ 0.11)
Mason et al. (4)	84	0.77	0.89	0.66 ($\pm$ 0.08)
Roitman, Jones and Sheffield (5)	46	0.80	0.87	0.67 ($\pm$ 0.12)
This report	96	0.59	0.94	0.53 ($\pm$ 0.08)

dicated by the Index of merit, is somewhat lower than in two other studies; this might be explained by the fact that we only examined patients with a normal electrocardiogram taken at rest. It has been shown, e.g. by the studies of Gensini (2), that these patients almost always show extensive collateralization, which of course could be responsible for a delayed ischemic response in the exercise test.

Although the GXT performed more satisfactorily than the step test, there was nevertheless a substantial number of false negative responders in the GXT: i.e. patients with a negative bicycle test but with marked coronary sclerosis. This fraction of false-negative responders appeared especially high among patients with isolated occlusions of the right coronary artery. In this study, there were eight cases with isolated occlusions of the right coronary artery, seven of them showing a negative GXT. This is of course too small a number to warrant statistical significance, but we think it likely that ischemia produced by coronary obstructions of the diaphragmatical myocardial wall is difficult to detect by these exercise tests.

REFERENCES

1. Van Herpen, G., Bruschke, A. V. G. & Hanssen, A. W., The correlation between the coronary arteriogram and other diagnostic parameters. *11th International Symposium on Vectorcardiography*. New York 1970.

2. Martinez-Rios, M. A., Bruto Da Costa, B. C., Cecena-Seldner, F. A. & Gensini, G. G., Normal electrocardiogram in the presence of severe coronary artery disease, *Amer. J. Cardiol.* 25, 320 (1970).

3. Kassebaum, D. G., Sutherland, K. I. & Judkins, M., A comparison of hypoxemia and exercise electrocardiography in coronary artery disease, *Amer. Heart J.* 75, 759 (1968).

4. Mason, R. E., Likar, I., Biern, R. O. & Ross, R. S., Multiple lead exercise electrocardiography, experience in 107 normal subjects with angina pectoris and comparison with coronary cine arteriography in 84 patients. *Circulation* 36, 517 (1967).

5. Roitman, D., Jones, W. B. & Sheffield, L. T., Comparison of submaximal exercise ECG test with coronary cine cardiogram, *Ann. intern. Med.* 72, 641 (1970).

QUANTITATIVE APPROACH TO EXERCISE TESTING FOR ISCHEMIC HEART DISEASE*

L. T. SHEFFIELD

SUMMARY

Application of dynamic and quantitative methods to exercise electrocardiography has lagged partly because of technical difficulties in acquiring exercise electrocardiographic signals and partly because of limitation imposed by the conventional means of ECG registration. Contemporary methods relieve these restrictions and permit changes in response to exercise stress to be measured as they occur, so that the time-course of response becomes a significant variable. This permits the adoption of an exercise stress method which becomes part of a closed feedback loop with individual response to exercise determining the cut off point of the stress. Such a stress test is shown to be reproducible to a satisfactory degree and effective in detecting ischemic heart disease.

A visual method for quantitating exercise ST segment response is illustrated. Its use will reduce interobserver variation in the evaluation of exercise ECGs. A computer method of processing exercise ECGs is described. It eliminates human variability in measurement as well as reducing physician time and effort requirements in evaluating exercise ECG response.

INTRODUCTION

The wide prevalence of ischemic heart disease in western civilizations has given impetus to many efforts aimed at the diagnosis, treatment and future prevention of this disease. Though in the past the clinician found it necessary to rely solely on skillful evaluation of symptom patterns for the diagnosis of angina pectoris, he now has available a wide variety of tests to aid his diagnosis. These tests occupy an entire spectrum in terms of diagnostic effectiveness, safety, availability and cost. They include the conven-

* Supported by Grant He-11310-03 of the U.S. Public Health Service, the Alabama Heart Association, and by Clinical Research Center Grant 5M01-FR-00032-10.

tional resting electrocardiogram, the stress electrocardiogram, kineto-cardiogram, systolic time interval measurement, stress thermogram, paced electrocardiogram, coronary sinus lactate measurement, ventriculographic measurement, coronary arteriograms and many others. Of all these tests and modes of examination, the exercise electrocardiogram has proved to be the most generally useful diagnostic aid in terms of sensitivity, specificity, avail-ability and safety. Application of quantitative techniques to this useful method has been somewhat delayed by the great variability of the disease process itself and by the graphic nature of the process used to record the electrical signal of the heart, which consequently gave rise to descriptive terms for alterations in this signal and a pictorial rather than numerical correlation between the electrocardiogram and the disease it was used to measure. Fortunately this situation has now changed to a considerable degree.

I. QUANTITATION OF STRESS

In their study of the relationship between exercise test response and ob-served life expectancy, Robb and Marks demonstrated a striking degree of excess mortality among persons with exertional ST segment depression (1). Conversely they found normal or decreased mortality associated with the absence of exercise ECG changes. In studying the electrocardiographic re-sponse to exercise of normal volunteers and patients with ischemic heart disease, we and others found that the conventional two-step exercise stress was frequently insufficient to provoke clinical or electrocardiographic manifestations of ischemia even though disease was known to be present (2, 3, 4). Further study indicated that more intense stress would uncover the abnormal finding in an increased percentage of patients. The initial fear that near maximal or maximal exercise stress would introduce false positive re-sponses by provoking 'physiologic' ischemia even in normal individuals was not substantiated (5). Maximal exercise stress is tolerated by normal persons of all ages without the production of symptoms or electrocardiographic changes suggestive of myocardial ischemia. The available evidence thus suggests that maximum exercise stress would provide more sensitive detec-tion of ischemic heart disease than would any lesser degree of stress. In spite of this there are some important arguments against the general use of maximum exercise stress in screening for ischemic heart disease. One is the anxiety a physician has that his patient who is sedentary, elderly or enduring some infirmity, might somehow undergo harm if he or she suddenly under-took to perform maximal exercise. Another difficulty with standardizing upon maximal exercise is the difficulty of recognizing effectively this level of performance when it is achieved (6). Since the degree of motivation will vary from patient to patient, the attainment of maximal exercise stress must be inferred from the demonstration that maximal oxygen consumption has been attained. This documentation adds considerable complexity to the exercise test procedure, so we sought a simpler and more readily acceptable means of standardizing exercise stress. As shown in figure I maximal exer-

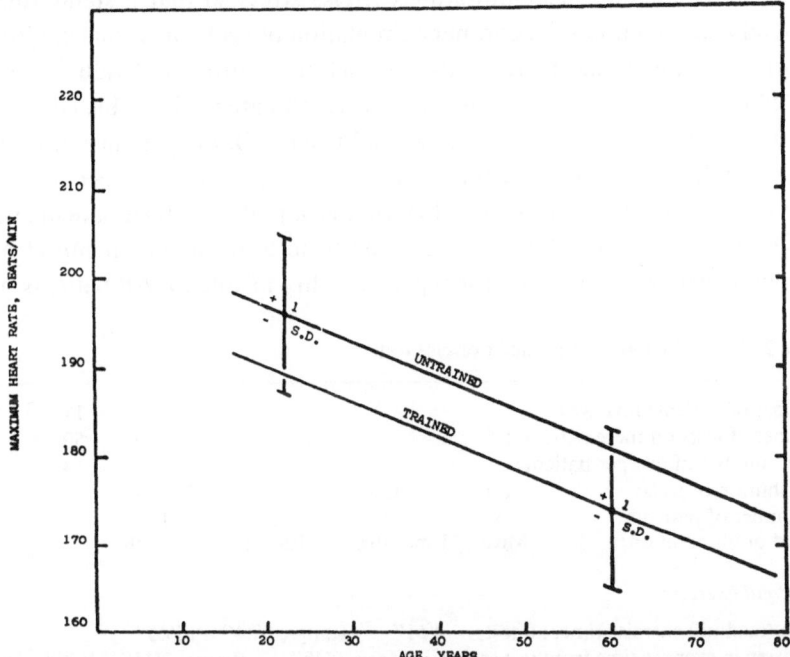

Fig. I. Maximum heart rate as a function of age and physical training, as determined in a wide age range of volunteer men, selected for their good health and cooperative spirit.

cise heart rate may be predicted on the basis of subject age and activity history (7). Since in the normal individual the heart rate response is the most significant single determinant of myocardial oxygen consumption changes during exercise, the attainment of a specified fraction, e.g. 90%, of maximal heart rate during exercise may be equated with a standardized demand for myocardial perfusion through the coronary arteries (Table I)*.

* It should be emphasized that the aimed-for exercise heart rate for each individual represents the exercise cut off point when no abnormality has been demonstrated during stress up to that point. In case any evidence of exercise intolerance is recognized, exercise is promptly terminated without regard for 'target heart rate'.

Table 1. Target heart rate for GXT.

Age	40	45	50	55	60	65	70
Untrained Subject	170	168	166	164	162	160	158
Regular Exercise ≥ 3/week	164	162	159	158	156	154	152

If the above method of quantitating exercise stress so that a standardized demand is placed upon the coronary circulation of each individual subject is a correct one, it should be reproducible such that normal individuals on repeated testing yield normal results, and diseased patients in stable condition repeatedly yield about the same abnormal results. Our experience in testing normal individuals confirms this with false positive findings occurring in only one to three percent of cases (8). In a group of seventeen patients with stable angina pectoris, fifty graded exercise tests recorded on initial and followup visits were analyzed for reproducibility (Table 2). All patients had

Table 2. Reproducibility of graded exercise test.

Number of patients reviewed:				17
Number of tests on these patients:				50
Mean number of test per patient:				3
Distribution of tests:	2 tests	3 tests	4 tests	5 tests
Number of patients:	8	3	5	1
Period of observation:	Mean, 7½ months		Range, 2-33 months	

Treadmill exercise

Mean treadmill exercise time, all tests: 4′51″   Range, 0′34″ – 10′45″
Variation in exercise time from test to test: Mean, 0′48″   Range, 0′14″ – 3′20″
Percentage variation in treadmill exercise time, 17%

Peak exercise heart rate

Mean exercise heart rate: 123.2/minute   Range, 88 – 168
Variation in heart rate from test to test: Mean, 6.62/minute   Range, 0 – 30/minute
Percentage variation in exercise heart rate: 5.4%

at least two tests, and one patient had a total of five tests performed over an interval of thirty-one months (Fig. 2). Using a standardized treadmill work schedule, the mean exercise time was four minutes fifty-one seconds, and the mean variation from one test to another on the same individual was forty-eight seconds. Mean test-retest treadmill exercise time variation was seventeen percent. During testing the peak exercise heart rate averaged 123 per minute for all tests, and the test-retest peak heart rate variation was 6.6 beats per minute. This is a 5.4% variation in heart rate for repeated testing of the same individual. These results indicate that the method is indeed quite

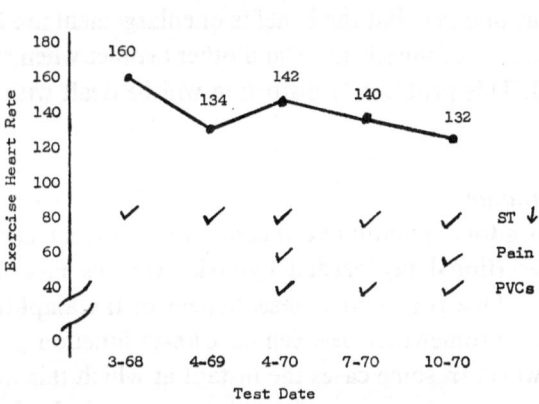

Patient B. C., 56 year old caucasian male

Fig. 2. Results of repeating Graded exercise test in a single patient. In each case exercise was discontinued when definite ischemic type s t depression was recognized while monitoring exercise. The peak exercise heart rate is plotted above. Check marks indicate the presence of s t depression, angina pectoris and ventricular premature beats for each test date.

reproducible. Further, they suggest that the test has value in following the course of ischemic heart disease and recognizing significant changes in severity of a patient's condition.

II. QUANTITATION OF ELECTROCARDIOGRAPHIC RESPONSE

Angina pectoris is by its very nature a paroxysmal affliction, and its electrocardiographic correlate has been classically recognized as a temporary negative displacement of the RS-T segment in an ECG lead positively oriented to the left ventricle. Other less specific ECG changes have been recorded in abundance, such as T wave inversion or other changes, ST segment elevation, and temporary appearance of ventricular or supraventricular arrhythmias and conduction disturbances. Fortunately these less specific findings are uncommon in patients with milder forms of ischemic heart disease in whom the diagnosis is relatively more difficult and the implications for modifying or ameliorating the disease presumably more promising.

Exercise electrocardiography and also other branches of this field have been hampered by the continued employment of the same recording format originally introduced, namely a chart speed of 25 mm/sec and a deflection sensitivity of 1 cm/mV. This format imposes a stringent limitation on the degree of precision which can be realized through visual interpretation of the record. Some laboratories have improved this situation by including at least one cardiac cycle recorded at high speed and sensitivity for improved wave form interpretation. Exercise electrocardiograms in particular would benefit from this practice, but the benefits of enlargement are largely neutralized by the presence of muscle noise and other artifact when strenuous exercise is involved. This problem of distortion will be dealt with in a later section.

A. Visual quantitation

In an effort to adopt quantitative measurements for ST segment changes attributed to exertional myocardial hypoxia, various measurements have been introduced. One is a simple measurement of the amplitude of ST segment displacement somewhere between the QRS-ST junction (J point) and the peak of the T wave. In some cases the instant at which this measurement is made has been specified, e.g. 40, 60 or 80 msec after the J point or after some fiducial point within the QRS complex itself. Since slope of the ST segment is important as well as its amplitude, and upsloping ST segments associated with J point depression have been recognized as normal, my colleagues and I initially sought to introduce quantitative measurement by specifying the amplitude of the J point in mV and the slope of the ST segment expressed in mV/sec (5). It was found that our patients with angina pectoris on exercise developed junctional depression equal or greater than 0.1 mV associated with an ST segment slope equal or less than plus 1 mV/sec. This measurement may be made readily on consecutive cardiac cycle having a stable baseline, and Dr. Herman K. Hellerstein has further simplified the measurement using a transparent overlay of his own design (Fig. 3) (9). It has been found repeatedly that when electrocardiographers interpret exercise records by visual inspection without performing careful measurement of individual cardiac cycles, there is a tremendous interobserver variation in the interpretation of identical records (10).

B. A computer method for measurement of exercise ECG response

Computer measurement of the exercise electrocardiogram suggests several possible advantages. The classical format of ECG recording may be dropped in favour of one which treats the heart signal as a time series of bits of pure information and not as a picture or graph. Measurements can be made

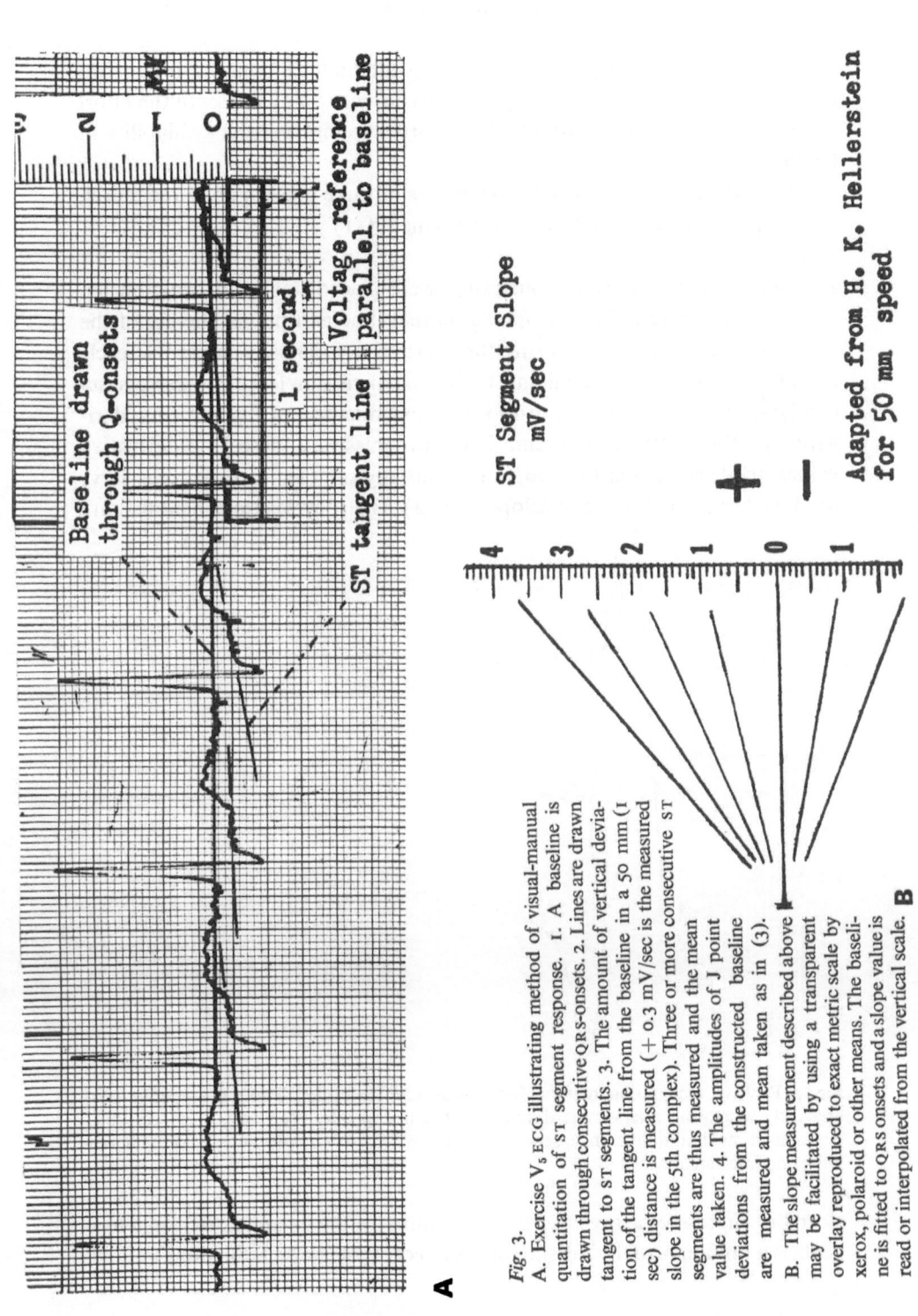

A

B

Fig. 3.
A. Exercise V₅ ECG illustrating method of visual-manual quantitation of ST segment response. 1. A baseline is drawn through consecutive QRS-onsets. 2. Lines are drawn tangent to ST segments. 3. The amount of vertical deviation of the tangent line from the baseline in a 50 mm (1 sec) distance is measured (+ 0.3 mV/sec is the measured slope in the 5th complex). Three or more consecutive ST segments are thus measured and the mean value taken. 4. The amplitudes of J point deviations from the constructed baseline are measured and mean taken as in (3).

B. The slope measurement described above may be facilitated by using a transparent overlay metric scale by xerox, polaroid or other means. The baseline is fitted to QRS onsets and a slope value is read or interpolated from the vertical scale.

with precision according to an unvarying method, eliminating interpreta-
tional inconstancy. Finally, computer measurement may conserve the effort
of the physician electrocardiographer in order to improve the availability of
health care.

The program we have developed consists of three phases: noise reduction,
wave form recognition and wave measurement (11).

1. Noise reduction: Certain constraints were placed upon our program because of our desire to have it operate in real time and permit the use of the
program as an aid in monitoring the exercise test. Thus each cardiac cycle
must be recognized after analogue to digital conversion (500 samples per second) using only a fast, forward looking examination of the first time derivative of the electrocardiogram. Three progressively increasing derivative
values, the least greater than 20% of an initially sampled cardiac cycle, serve
to identify each R wave downslope (Fig. 4). Heart cycles thus identified are

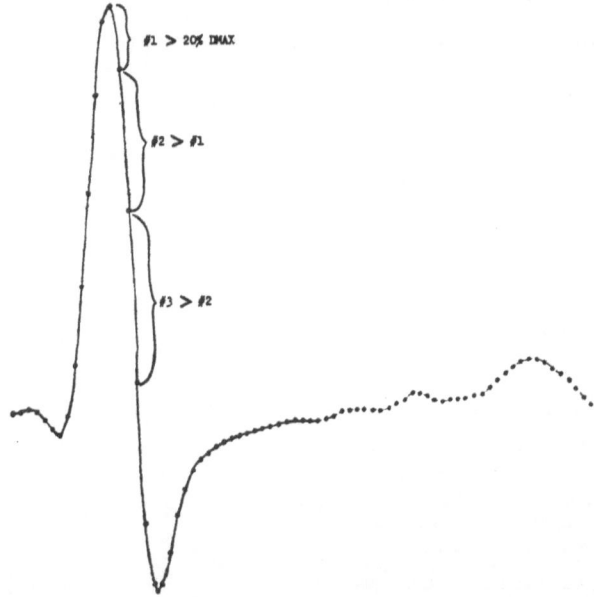

Fig. 4. R wave recognition method for storing cardiac cycles. Three consecutive progressively increasing intersample differences, the first greater than 20% of a previously
determined maximum difference, serve to recognize the QRS complex in spite of moderate
noise and interference.

stored in successive arrays. A variable number of beats are stored; nineteen
beats is a number usually satisfactory for acceptable noise reduction. Follow-

ing storage of the nineteenth beat, a point by point arithmetic median complex is constructed to represent this ECG sample. The process of median extraction reduces noise in a way similar to averaging but with the additional advantage of complete immunity to occasional large transient noise values.

2. *Wave form recognition:* From the calculated median complex a running first time derivative is calculated, and this is examined in a forward and backward fashion to recognize QRS onset, R peak, S nadir, J point, T peak and T end. The entire cardiac cycle is justified to zero amplitude at the recognized instant of QRS onset, and other amplitudes are measured accordingly. The instant of ST segment zero crossing, when present, is identified.

3. *Wave measurement:* All the points mentioned undergo amplitude measurement, the intervals between any two recognized points are measured, and area measurement or voltage-time integration is performed on the ST and T regions. We reasoned that in preference to a single instantaneous measurement of ST segment amplitude a more valuable figure would be one representative of the entire time course of the ST segment, hence the area or integral measurement. The T wave was treated similarly.

C. Computer outputs

Outputs from this program are designed to serve three purposes. These are to provide 1. timely 'on-line' feedback to the exercise laboratory for aid in monitoring the exercising subject, 2. a printed record of measurements for the subject's medical record, and 3. a record of all this information on digital magnetic tape for subsequent 'off-line' evaluation in connection with research projects.

Real time outputs to the exercise laboratory include a beat-recognition pulse simultaneous with the storage of each heart cycle, which may be used to flash a light or otherwise assure the investigator that the program input is operating. A set of outputs for a storage oscilloscope automatically erase the screen and trace the current median complex inclusing identification of the various waves as recognized (Fig. 5); and finally, a teletype output which after each ECG sample immediately writes the time, heart rate and all the programmed ECG measurements. On our PDP-7/9 computer these measurements are reported 2.5 to 4 seconds following the last beat of an ECG sample. At this time the digital median complex and all the measurements are recorded on a block of magnetic tape. In the course of the exercise test this process is recycled continually about four times per minute, depending on the heart rate. It also continues during the postexercise recovery period.

Following termination of recording, the digital tape is automatically rewound and examined under program control for the production of an exercise test summary sheet by a digital plotter. Samples are automatically

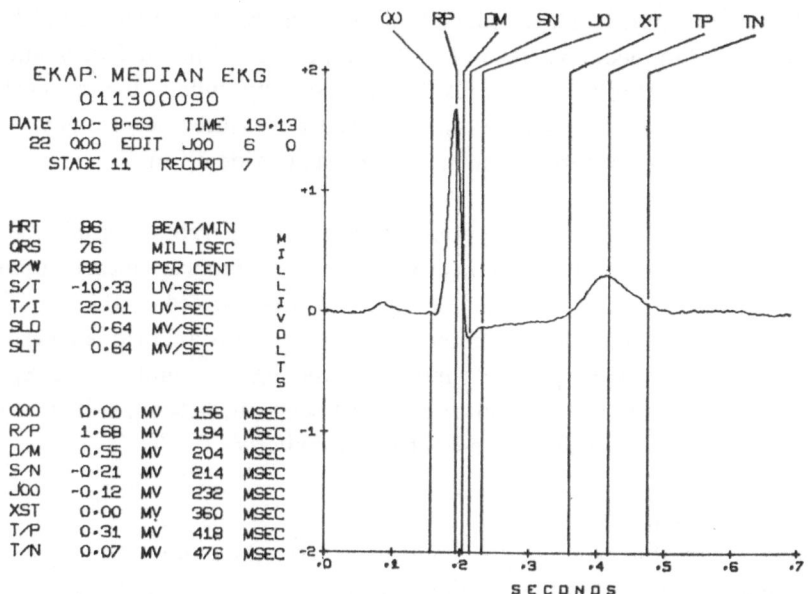

Fig. 5. Wave form recognition and measurement: computer generated display for monitor scope and digital plotter. Wave form display at right and measurements on left. Upper left: identification data; left center: rate, duration, amplitude and area measurements. Lower left: temporal location of each recognition.

selected from the beginning of exercise, midexercise, peak exercise, initial recovery period and late recovery period, and these are drawn by the plotter along with selected measurements of each. Finally, a graph of the ST segment integral with respect to heart rate is plotted to permit visual appreciation of the dynamic behavior of the ST segment during exercise and subsequent rest (Fig. 6).

III. CLINICAL RESULTS

Computer measurement of the graded exercise test electrocardiogram was evaluated by testing a group of forty-one clinically normal men and a group of thirty-eight patients of comparable mean age (12). Each of the thirty-eight patients had a history of episodes of squeezing or expanding substernal chest discomfort brought on by exertion, meals and/or cold exposure lasting two to ten minutes and promptly relieved by rest or nitroglycerin. Progressive treadmill exercise was carried out until some evidence of abnormality was appreciated or until the target heart rate, 90% of predicted maximum exercise

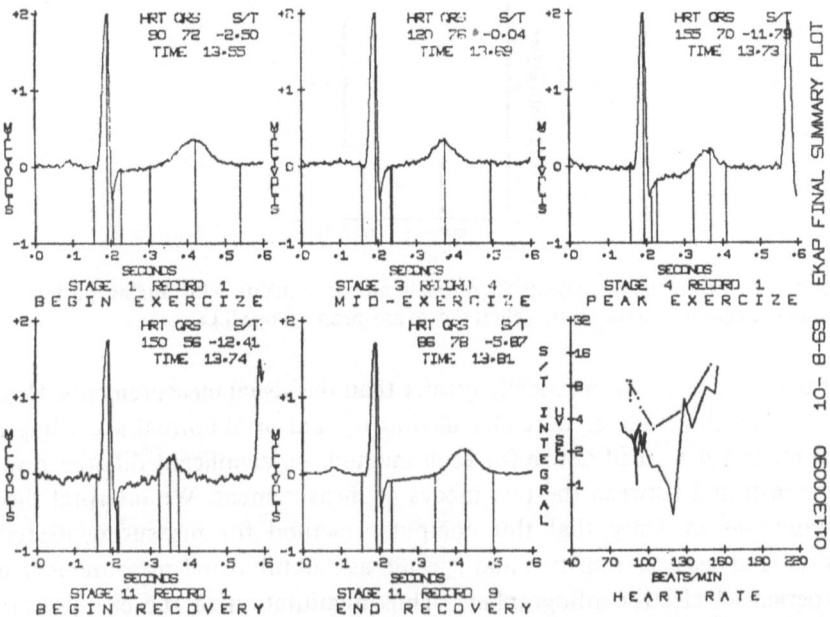

Fig. 6. Exercise test summary sheet, composed and plotted by program control. Above are shown, left to right, V_5 ECG at beginning of exercise, midexercise and peak exercise. Below are initial and late postexercise records and a graph of ST segment response with respect to heart rate (interrupted part of curve indicates postexercise measurement).

heart rate, was reached for each person. The V_5 electrocardiogram was recorded on magnetic tape and processed by computer. The normal group was found to have ST integral measurements with an exercise mean value of 4.3 ± 2.9 μVsec (± 1 S.D.). Exercise ST value for angina pectoris patients was 15.3 ± 8.2 μVsec (± 1 S.D.) (Fig. 7). On the basis of these findings a normal range of zero to − 7.5 μVsec was tentatively adopted. Later Dr. C. P. Riley and Dr. Albert Oberman in cooperation with the writer subjected seventy graded exercise test V_5 electrocardiograms to careful visual measurement as prescribed by the Minnesota Code (13) and compared these measurements with computer measurements made by our program on the same electrocardiograms (14). Of these seventy tests, thirty-five demonstrated ST segment depression equal to or greater than 0.1 mV with a flat or negative slope, and thirty-five tests demonstrated lesser degrees of change or none at all. The results of visual measurement and of computer measurement were subjected to statistical analysis, and as expected the computer measurements of

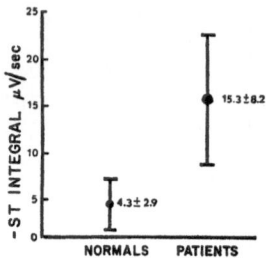

Fig. 7. ST integral measurements in normals and in patients with angina pectoris, in response to graded exercise test. Values shown are means $\pm$ one S.D.

ST segments were systematically greater than the visual measurements. However when the readings were classified as normal or abnormal according to the criteria described above for each method, no significant difference was demonstrated between the two modes of measurement. We interpret these findings as evidence that this computer method for measuring exercise ECGs is at least as sensitive and specific as careful visual measurement by experienced electrocardiographers. Thus quantitation of the exercise ECG appears indeed to have been realized. Only future experience can show what benefit it may have for cardiovascular research and practice.

REFERENCES

1. Robb, G. P. & Marks, H. H., Latent coronary artery disease: determination of its presence and severity by the exercise electrocardiogram. *Amer. J. Cardiol.* 13, 603 (1964).
2. Sheffield, L. T. & Reeves, T. J., Graded exercise in the diagnosis of angina pectoris. *Mod. Conc. cardiov. Dis.* 34, 1 (1965).
3. Friedberg, C. K., Jaffe, H. L., Pordy, L. & Chesky, K., The two-step exercise electrocardiogram. A double-blind evaluation of its use in the diagnosis of angina pectoris. *Circulation* 26, 1254 (1962).
4. Rowell, L. B., Taylor, H. L., Simonson, E. & Carlson, W. S., The physiologic fallacy of adjusting for body weight in performance of the Master two-step test. *Amer. Heart J.* 70, 461 (1965).
5. Lester, F. M., Sheffield, L. T. & Reeves, T. J., Electrocardiographic changes in clinically normal older men following near maximal and maximal exercise. *Circulation* 36, 5 (1967).

6. Hermiston, R. T. & Faulkner, J. A., Prediction of maximal oxygen uptake by a step-wise regression technique. *J. appl. Physiol.* 30, 883 (1971).
7. Lester, M., Sheffield, L. T., Trammell, P. & Reeves, T. J., The effect of age and athletic training on the maximal heart rate during muscular exercise. *Amer. Heart J.* 76, 370 (1968).
8. Sheffield, L. T., Holt, J. H. & Reeves, T. J., Exercise graded by heart rate in electro-cardiographic testing for angina pectoris. *Circulation* 32, 622 (1965).
9. Hellerstein, H. K., Exercise therapy in coronary disease. *Bull. N. Y. Acad. Med.* 44, 1028 (1968).
10. Blackburn, H., et al., The exercise electrocardiogram: Differences in interpretation. Report of a technical group on exercise electrocardiography. *Amer. J. Cardiol.* 21, 871 (1968).
11. Sheffield, L. T., Conroy, D. V., Holt, J. H., Lester, F. M. & Reeves, T. J., Diagnosis of coronary artery disease by on-line computer processing of the exercise electrocardiogram. *Proceedings of the 21st Annual Conference on Engineering in Medicine and Biology*, p. 40.1, November 1968.
12. Sheffield, L. T., Holt, J. H., Lester, F. M., Conroy, D. V. & Reeves, T. J., On-line analysis of the exercise electrocardiogram. *Circulation* 40, 935 (1969).
13. Blackburn, H., Keys, A., Simonson, E., Rautaharju, P. & Punsar, S., The electrocardiogram in population studies – A classification system. *Circulation* 31, 1160 (1960).
14. Riley, C. P., Oberman, A. & Sheffield, L. T., Unpublished data.

DISCUSSION

Varnauskas: Ischaemic ECG changes and anginal pain are believed to occur when myocardial oxygen demands exceed oxygen supply. Consequently in evaluating coronary reserve the appropriate variables of ischaemia should be related to the determinants of myocardial oxygen demand.

There are four major determinants of myocardial oxygen demand: heart rate, blood pressure, heart volume (blood pressure and heart volume are the major determinants of wall tension) and myocardial contractility. Two, heart rate and systolic blood pressure, can be readily measured in clinical practice and by laboratory procedures.

It has been demonstrated that changes in the product of heart rate times systolic blood pressure (HR × SBP) provide a reasonably close approximation of an over-all change in myocardial oxygen demand, if the testing conditions do not provoke significant alterations in either heart volume or exclusive contractility of the myocardium. The appearance of angina pectoris and/or ischaemic ECG changes during physical exercise, and pacing-induced tachycardia shows better correlation with the product HR × SBP than with HR or BP alone, in an individual patient with stable coronary heart disease. Heart rate and systolic blood pressure response to a given exercise load can vary considerably from time to time. Consequently the levels of heart rate, or systolic blood pressure, provoking angina pectoris can differ considerably for two or more consecutive tests. Combining the heart rate and systolic blood pressure into the product HR × SBP offers a more reliable index of the mechanical load on the heart (or myocardial oxygen demand) which causes angina pectoris.

Furthermore it has been shown that the correlation between coronary flow and HR × SBP is linear up to a fourfold increase in these variables produced by exercise in subjects with normal coronary circulation. However, in patients with coronary heart disease the increase in coronary flow caused by exercise levels off with respect to the increase in HR × SBP. If heart rate alone is used instead of the product, the resulting correlation with coronary flow is linear in both patients and normal individuals, i.e. it does not differentiate between coronary heart diseased patients and subjects with normal coronary circulation.

Gradually induced tachycardia using the atrial pacing technique is a stress procedure frequently used to test coronary reserve. However, pacing-induced tachycardia does not always provoke symptoms and signs of myocardial ischaemia. This is due to the fact that such an increase in heart rate, even to high values, causes only a moderate increase in myocardial oxygen demand and requires less increase in coronary flow than exercise. A significant increase in systolic blood pressure during pacing is absent. The maximum value of HR × SBP achieved by pacing is always less than the maximum obtained by exercise. The lack of increase in systolic blood pressure, as well as the reduced rise in contractility, during pacing in contrast to exercise explains the difference between exercise and pacing tests.

In conclusion the tests imposing the largest possible mechanical load and thus the largest possible oxygen demand on the myocardium are superior in disclosing ischaemia and in testing coronary reserve, especially in patients with moderate impairment of coronary circulation.

Sheffield: There are two things that I would like to mention. First I am very glad that the difference between the heart rate response with pacing and the heart rate response with exercise was brought out because this fits in so beautifully with the way people tend to explain how the heart works and why exercise tests work. The thing which I cannot agree with is the choice of a single lead for exercise testing. If we have a test that is less than 90% sensitive even at its best, are we willing to sacrifice 5, 6 or 8% of that simply by making the test a little bit easier or a little bit quicker or a little bit cheaper? It has been proved I believe beyond dispute – Blackburn for example has examined lead sensitivity with ST segment changes – that there are some ST changes that occur in the longitudinal direction of the body which cannot be picked up by lead 1 or lead V5 or V6 but will be picked up by using a longitudinally sensitive lead. There are other times but not as frequent, perhaps 2% but at least 1-2%, when the change is directed in anteroposterior direction. In this case a lead which does not have sensitivity in the front-back direction is going to miss it. That is the reason we record one lead that is directed transversely (V5), one lead that is directed front-back and one lead longitudinally (AVF), or we use the Frank XYZ system.

Ascoop: I agree with Dr. Sheffield about the XYZ system. We used a Frank system because all the information can be included in only 3 leads and this is an important feature in data reduction for automatic processing.

Snellen: Could Dr. Denolin give his comments, in particular about the other parameters of the exercise test and the effect of training?

Denolin: Our study on the effect of muscular training after myocardial infarction was conducted following a protocol accepted by several laboratories under the direction of Bruce from Seattle. All together we studied 12 patients 40-60 years old, 2-4 months after the myocardial infarction without cardiac failure and without cardiotonic or β blocking drugs. Before training all patients were tested on a bicycle ergometer. In the first study our aim was a maximum exercise test. In a group of 7 patients we were able to obtain a truly maximum oxygen consumption, but in a second group the patients were stopped by pain or exhaustion. The day after the first maximum tests we took a submaximum test at 40% and 70% of the maximum with measurement of oxygen consumption, the arterial pressure, cardiac output, ECG, lactic acid, P_{O_2} and P_{CO_2} in arterial blood. After these two tests training with 3 times a week began 25 minutes of exercise at 40% of maximum during the first week, then 70% during the second week and for the last 5 weeks 90% of the maximum. The following conclusion could be made: A training of 25 minutes 3 times a week is sufficient to increase the maximal work capacity of the patients on the condition that the level of training represents an important part of the aerobic capacity. In that case we can observe a decrease in heart rate or a decrease in the ventricular volume without any changes in the total cardiac output. In all cases we saw some peripheral changes, such as an important decrease in lactic acid, for the same amount of work.

Snellen: I think Dr. Sheffield has had some experience in the prognostic significance of the success of training.

Sheffield: Among the patients who were trained there was a minority in whom the work capacity and heart rate did not change. These patients had a high mortality. Several died in the interval between recommending coronary bypass surgery and the time that surgery was actually scheduled. Now we consider this lack of reaction to training as a semi-emergency indication for operation.

Pool: We have also had some experience in training cardiac patients and I agree with Dr. Sheffield that some patients with a low maximum heart rate show a poor training result and also a high mortality. However, our figures are too small to be significant.

Van Herpen: I have a question for Dr. Varnauskas. He told us that oxygen consumption 'when plotted against heart rate' did not offer any discrimination between normal individuals and patients with coronary sclerosis. On the other hand differentiation is possible using the product of systolic blood pressure times heart rate. I wonder whether you might not drop heart rate from this formula; mathematically you could use systolic blood pressure alone.

Varnauskas: In this material it was not so simple. Systolic blood pressure did not differentiate significantly, although there was some difference between patients and controls. Combined heart rate and pressure did provide a differentiation. We should include more factors which determine the oxygen demand of the myocardium rather than drop them.

CHAPTER 3

PERIPHERAL CIRCULATION

QUANTITATIVE MEASUREMENTS OF BLOOD FLOW
AND BLOOD PRESSURE IN MUSCLE AND SKIN

O. A. LARSEN AND G. BELL

Patients with occlusions of the arteries to the lower extremities can be separated clinically and pathophysiologically into two main groups: 1. patients with pains on exertion as the cardinal symptom and 2. patients who also have ischaemic pains at rest and eventually develop chronic gangrene.

In patients with intermittent claudication, the distal arterial blood pressure (i.e. the local perfusion pressure) is practically normal at rest, but the collateral vessels can not maintain this pressure when the arteriolar tone decreases during muscular exercise. These patients have *an intermittent distal hypotension.*

In patients with severe occlusions of the arteries to the legs and an underdeveloped collateral circulation, the local perfusion pressure will be low in the distal vascular areas, even at rest. Thus these patients have *a permanent distal hypotension.*

For most of the patients with symptoms of peripheral circulatory disease, especially those with rest pains, one must today insist that relevant quantitative circulatory studies be performed. One requirement for an exact diagnosis and an evaluation of the various treatments given these patients is that the blood flow and/or the blood pressure be measured at the right place and at the right time. We would like to stress the importance of measuring the distal arterial blood pressure. Just as one obviously measures the systemic blood pressure in a patient in shock, then too just as obviously one should measure distal pressure in occlusive vascular disease, which as such merely constitutes a condition of local shock.

Blood flow and blood pressure in peripheral muscles and skin can be measured using the local tissue clearance technique with radioactive xenon as the indicator. The tests mentioned below are easily and rapidly performed and include no risk to the patients.

* This study was supported by a grant from 'The King Christian X Foundation'.

In patients with intermittent claudication as the cardinal symptom our routine investigation is the:

XENON-I 33 STANDARDIZED WALKING TEST (I, 2).

Procedure: 0.1 ml of ^{133}Xe dissolved in isotonic saline (0.5-1.0 mCi per milliliter) is injected with a thin needle (0.4 mm outer diameter) into the thickest part of the medial head of the gastrocnemius muscle. Care is taken that no gas bubbles are injected (flush through needle before injecting) and that none of the xenon solution is deposited in tissues other than the muscle. A similar injection is given in the opposite leg.

Two small scintillation probes, weighing only 80 grams each, are attached medially and anteriorly to the leg by adhesive tape. The detector crystals are placed as accurately as possible on the surface of the skin over the intramuscular depots. Care must be taken not to apply the tape too tightly, or circulation in the muscle may be hampered.

A coaxial cable, several meters long, is attached between the probe and a charge-sensitive amplifier, allowing the patient considerable freedom of movement. Each amplifier is coupled to a scaler with a time constant of 5 seconds and to a logarithmic potentiometer writer (paper speed 10 mm/min). The maximum counting rate is normally about 3000 counts per second.

Following injection of the isotope, the subject stands motionless on a treadmill for 3 to 5 minutes, while the resting muscle clearance is registered. The treadmill used in our walking test has a speed of 4.5 km/hr. The elevation of the treadmill is either 8% or 16% and patients should be tested using the steepest grade on which they can walk for 1.5 to 2 minutes.

The patient walks until fatigue and pain in the legs stop him, usually after 2 minutes. The patient should walk as normally as possible and wear ordinary low-heeled walking shoes. Subjects not manifesting claudication are stopped after 5 to 10 minutes. After the walking test the patient stands motionless on the treadmill until the hyperemic phase passes and a slow, fairly constant clearance rate approximating the pre-exercise resting value has become established.

Calculations: When evaluating the ^{133}Xe clearance curve obtained during and after walking, it is easy upon immediate inspection of the curve to differentiate between a normal subject and a patient with an occlusive arterial disease: normal man has a marked calf muscle hyperemia during walking and the flow returns to the resting value within 1 to 2 min after cessation of walking. The patients with intermittent claudication show insufficient muscle blood flow during walking and a prolonged post-exercise hyperemic reaction (Fig. 1). Only haemodynamically significant arterial abnormalities can

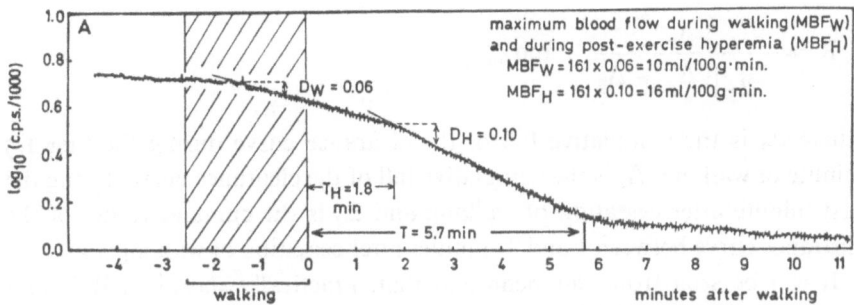

Fig. 1. A ^{133}Xe clearance curve obtained during and after the standardized walking test in a leg with an occlusion of the femoral artery. The curve shows a low blood flow for walking (MBFw in normal man is $>$ 10 ml/100 g . min) and higher blood flow after cessation of walking (in normal man MBF$_H$ never exceeds the value obtained for MBFw). T$_H$, the time from the cessation of walking to the commencement of MBF$_H$, is 1.8 min on this curve (T$_H$ is 0 min in normal man) and the total duration of post-walking hyperemia, T is 5.7 min (the upper normal limit for T is 3 min).

produce pathological post-exercise hyperemias, and the test clearly shows whether these pathological hyperemias are present.

A more objective evaluation of the ^{133}Xe clearance curve can be obtained by utilizing the following parameters.

1. Maximum muscle blood flow during walking (MBF$_W$).

MBF$_W$ = 100 $\cdot$ λ $\cdot$ ln(10) $\cdot$ D$_W$ml/100g $\cdot$ min = 161 $\cdot$ D$_W$ml/100g $\cdot$ min, where D$_W$ is the steepest slope of the tangent to the logarithmic clearance curve during walking.

2. Maximum muscle blood flow during the post-exercise hyperemia (MBF$_H$). MBF$_H$ = 161 $\cdot$ D$_H$ ml/100g $\cdot$ min, where D$_H$ is the steepest slope of the tangent to the logarithmic clearance curve during the post-exercise hyperemia.

3. Duration of the post-exercise hyperemia (T) measured in minutes. T is that time interval beginning with the cessation of walking and lasting until the muscle blood flow returns to a low and fairly constant value (the resting blood flow).

4. Time in minutes (T$_H$) between the end of walking and the beginning of MBF$_H$. T$_H$ is that time interval beginning with the cessation of walking and lasting until the post-exercise muscle blood flow (as indicated by the slope of the clearance curve) reaches its maximum value (steepest slope).

5. Index (R) for that part of the hyperemic reaction to exercise still remaining 1 min after cessation of walking.

This remaining hyperemia is calculated from the equation:

$$R = \frac{\Delta_3}{\Delta_1 + \Delta_2 + \Delta_3} \cdot 100\%,$$

where Δ_1 is the cumulative fall of the clearance curve during the first 1.5 minute of walking, Δ_2 is the cumulative fall of the clearance curve during the first minute after cessation of walking and Δ_3 is the cumulative fall of the clearance curve between 1 and T minutes after cessation of walking.

It can be seen from this definition that, practically speaking, R is that percentage of the total fall of the clearance curve which occurs after 1 minute of rest.

Results: The normal values of this test are given below.

MBF_W: Clinically the lowest limit of the norm is taken to be 10 ml/100g · min.

MBF_H: This value will never exceed the value obtained for MBF_W.

T: Clinically the highest limit of the norm is taken to be 3.0 min.

T_H: In normal man T_H is always 0 minutes, but due to technical problems (change in geometry) a value less than 1.0 min is taken as normal.

R: The value for the remaining hyperemia is less than 25% in normal subjects.

Clinical classifications: Normal response (legs may have mild to moderate but clinically insignificant stenosis in the femoral and/or iliac (common and external) artery): MBF_W = 10-40 ml/100 g · min; T = 0-3.0 min; T_H = 0-1.0 min and R = 0-25%.

Legs with either 1. total occlusion of the femoral artery with insignificant changes proximally, or 2. significant stenosis (subtotal obliteration) of the femoral and/or iliac (common and external) artery: MBF_W = 0-12 ml/100 g · min; T = more than 3.0 min; T_H = 0.0-4.0 min and R = 26 or about 90%.

Legs with occlusion of the femoral artery as well as either 1. total occlusion or 2. severe subtotal stenosis in the common and/or external iliac artery: MBF_W = 0-5 ml/100 g · min; T = more than about 9.0 min; T_H more than about 4.0 min and R = about 90-100%.

Comments: The ^{133}Xe walking test is easily and rapidly performed. The

Table 1. Xenon-133 ischaemia and exercise test. The interpretation of the laboratory results as sent to the clinical departments.

T min	MBF$_{max}$ ml/100 g.min	Diagnosis
< 0.8	> 60	Normal function of main arteries of the leg down to the level of the knee.
	35-60	* Normal function of main arteries of the leg down to the level of the knee is very likely: very rarely do cases with total or subtotal arterial occlusion above this level and with good collateral function show such results.
	< 35	Either obliterative disease of main arteries to the leg, usually without total obstruction and often causing no symptoms, or neuromuscular disease with normally functioning vessels.
0.8-2.0	> 35	* Total subtotal occlusion of main artery of the leg with good function of collateral vessels is most likely; in rare cases also found in younger normal individuals.
	15-35	Total or subtotal occlusion of main artery of the leg with some functioning collateral vessels.
	< 15	Total or subtotal occlusion of main artery of the leg with poor function of collateral vessels.
> 2.0	> 35	Occlusion of main artery of the leg with good function of collateral vessels.
	15-35	Occlusion of main artery of the leg with some function of collateral vessels.
	< 15	Occlusion of main artery of the leg with poor function of collateral vessels.

* The values for normal individuals and diseased subjects overlap by several percent.

entire test including calculations requires 30 minutes and can be performed by a nurse or technician. Risk to patients and personnel is almost non-existent. No complications whatsoever have been seen in over 2000 routine examinations using the test. Practically all the ^{133}Xe is eliminated from the body through the lungs during the isotope's first passage through the pulmonary circulation, with the result that radiation dosages to the patients are minimal. Gonadal radiation doses for a single test are 1/10,000 of the dose of a single x-ray film over the pelvis.

Deviations do occur in the clearance curves. They are due to limb movement with consequent alteration of the probe's counting geometry; they are very easy to recognize and correct. Erroneous injection of the isotope into non-muscular tissue is probably responsible for the rare occurrence (1-2% of curves) of a very small ^{133}Xe wash-out response not seen again on repeated retesting. This type of curve is readily recognized by the low amplitude of the cumulative clearance in the entire curve. To evaluate the post-exercise hyperemia it is important that the patient stand motionless on the treadmill after the walking period; if the muscles are truly at rest after walking, a post-exercise hyperemia can only be due to muscular ischaemia during exercise.

In special cases with occlusions in the distal arteries of the leg it may be preferable to inject the ^{133}Xe in calf muscles other than the medial gastrocnemius (e.g. lateral gastrocnemius, soleus or anterior tibial).

The following case history illustrates how quantitative flow measurements can provide a diagnosis in a suspected case of peripheral arterial disease.

Case 1. A 48 years old male complained of pain in both calves during exercise over the past year. On clinical examination all peripheral pulses, except the posterior tibial, were present. The patient had no ischaemic pain at rest and there were no skin changes consistent with arterial insufficiency. The Xenon-133 ischaemia and exercise test (see below) performed in the anterior tibial muscle was normal for both legs, indicating that there were no haemodynamically important stenoses in the arteries proximal to the muscle tissue under study.

However since the clinical symptoms were typical of intermittent claudication, a Xenon-133 walking test was performed. For the first test the isotope was injected into the anterior tibial muscles of both legs and for the second test, into the medial head of the gastrocnemius muscles (fig. 2). It can be seen from the figure that the walking test was normal for the anterior tibial group of muscles. The maximum blood flow during walking was within the normal range on both the right and left sides and after cessation of walking on the treadmill, the blood flow on both sides returned to the resting value within 3 minutes. However, when the test was repeated in the gastrocnemius muscles a different picture was seen. The blood flow increased during walking but the maximal blood flow did not occur until after walking had stopped, and the resting clearance was not re-established until 6 minutes after cessation of walking. This result is clearly abnormal and therefore an arteriogram was carried out. This showed bilateral occlusion of the posterior tibial artery, confirming the findings of the Xenon-133 walking test.

Thus the case demonstrates that the test can be normal for one group of calf muscles but abnormal for another; the test is therefore sensitive enough to provide a diagnosis of branch thrombosis.

In patients with intermittent claudication who cannot walk on the treadmill, we measure the muscle blood flow in the anterior tibial muscle after 5 minutes of ischemia using a blood pressure cuff, and exercise with the foot until exhaustion: the

XENON-133 ISCHAEMIA AND EXERCISE TEST (3, 4).

Procedure: The patient lies supine on a coach with the legs at heart level for at least 15 minutes before beginning the examination.

0.1 ml of ^{133}Xe dissolved in isotonic saline (0.5-1.0 mCi/ml) is injected with a thin needle (0.4 mm outer diameter) into the thickest part of the anterior tibial muscle. Care is taken that no gas bubbles are injected (flush

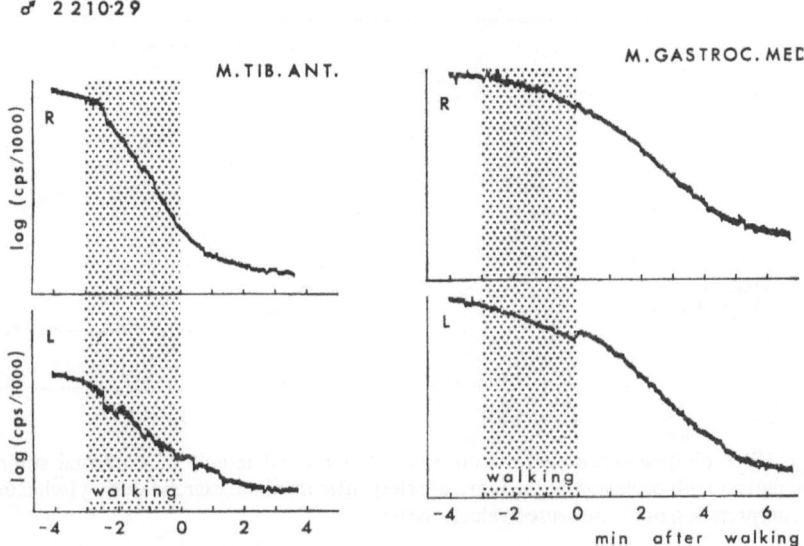

Fig. 2. The Xenon-133 walking test performed in a patient with a branch thrombosis of the posterior tibial artery. The isotope has been injected into the anterior tibial muscle (left) and medial gastrocnemius muscle (right). (For further details, see text).

through needle before injecting) and that none of the xenon solution is deposited in tissues other than the muscle. A similar injection is given in the opposite leg.

A blood pressure cuff (13 cm broad) is placed around each thigh. Two scintillation crystals (e.g. 1 × 1 inch NaI (Tl) crystals with photomultipliers) are placed about 10 cm from the skin. A collimator covering an area about 10 cm in diameter is used. Each crystal is coupled to a rate meter with a time constant of two seconds and the output from the rate meter is recorded on a logarithmic potentiometer writer with a paper speed of 10 mm per minute. The maximum counting rate is normally about 3000 counts per second.

The resting clearance rate is measured for 5 minutes. Then an arterial compression, applied by inflating the femoral cuffs to a pressure well above the systolic blood pressure (200-250 mm Hg), is maintained for 5 minutes.

During ischaemia the patients are asked to move their feet up and down using only the crural muscles (most patients can perform such movements at the ankle joint about 80-100 times). After exactly 5 minutes of ischaemia the cuffs are suddenly released, and during the subsequent stage of reactive hyperemia the ^{133}Xe clearance is followed for 5 to 10 minutes (Fig. 3).

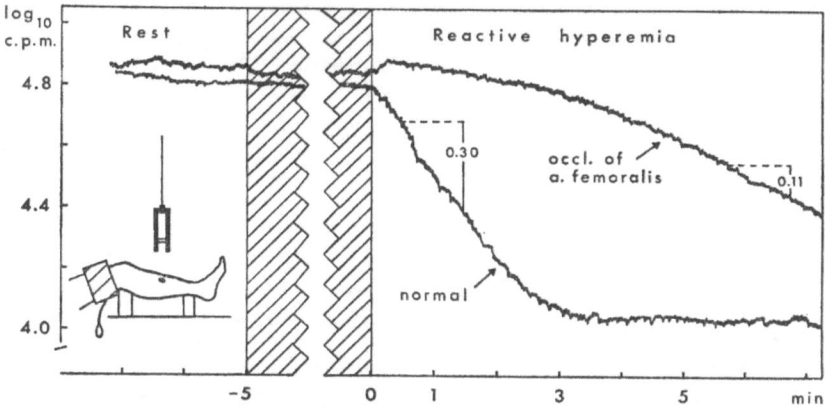

Fig. 3. [133]Xe disappearance curves from the anterior tibial muscle of a normal subject and a patient with occlusion of the femoral artery after maximal exercise during ischaemia (for interpretation of the measured values, see text).

Calculations: The maximum muscle blood flow (MBF) can be defined as:
MBF $=$ 100 $\cdot$ λ $\cdot$ ln(10) $\cdot$ D ml/100 g $\cdot$ min $=$ 161 $\cdot$ D ml/100 g $\cdot$ min, where D is the steepest slope of the tangent to the logarithmic clearance curve, measured as that fraction of a decade which the tangent decreases in one minute.

T is the time from the release of the arterial compression to the attainment of the maximum clearance rate.

Results: Normal values: for this technique the lowest value for the maximum muscle blood flow in the anterior tibial muscle is 35 ml/100 g $\cdot$ min (MBF averages 54.9 ml/100 g $\cdot$ min (SD $=$ 11.6 ml/100 g $\cdot$ min)).

The upper limit of the time to maximum blood flow is 0.8 minutes in normal individuals (T is on the average 0.37 min (SD $=$ 0.15)).

Clinical values: The two parameters measured provide different information. The longer the time between release of the arterial compression and attainment of MBF, the more severe the arterial occlusion. A localized stenosis gives a shorter T than a widespread total occlusion. The greater the maximum blood flow, the better the collateral circulation. Table I shows the interpretation of the laboratory results as sent to the clinical departments.

Comments: The ^{133}Xe ischaemia and exercise test requires about 30 minutes and can be performed by a nurse or technician. In patients operated on for occlusive vascular disease just above the knee or in the popliteal fossa, the cuff can be placed below the knee. The coefficient of variation in the maximal value of MBF is about 20%.

The study should always be repeated (possibly by covering the first injection site with a lead plate 4 cm in diameter and 2 mm thick) if: 1) unexpected results are found, 2) borderline results are found or 3) inadequate exercise of the anterior tibial muscle or partial injection of the indicator outside the muscle tissue is indicated by a curve which returns from hyperemia to resting values after less than 70% of the injected depot has been cleared.

Patients with severe arterial occlusions causing ischaemic pains at rest have a distal vascular bed where the arterioles are without tone, and yet – because of the low driving pressure – blood flow to the distal skin and muscles is also very low. In these patients the distal blood flow and the distal blood pressure can be measured using the
XENON-133 HISTAMINE TEST (5, 6, 7).

Procedure: 0.1 ml of a mixture of histamine and ^{133}Xe dissolved in isotonic saline (0.2 mg histamine chloride per 1 ml (1 mCi) ^{133}Xe in saline solution) is injected with a thin needle (0.4 mm outer diameter) into the skin of the dorsum of the foot producing a small papule. Care is taken that no gas bubbles are injected (flush through needle before injecting) and that none of the isotope-histamine solution is deposited in the subcutaneous tissue. A blood pressure cuff (13 cm broad) is placed around the foot, covering the isotope-histamine depot. The patient lies comfortably on a coach in supine position with the foot at heart level.

A scintillation crystal (e.g. a 1 × 1 inch NaI(Tl) crystal) is placed 5-10 cm from the foot directed tangentially toward the depot. The crystal is connected to a photomultiplier and coupled to a scaler with a time constant of two seconds. The output from the scaler is recorded on a logarithmic potentiometer writer with a paper speed of 10 mm per minute. The maximum counting rate is normally about 3000 counts per second.

Following injection of the isotope-histamine solution the patient lies motionless, while the clearance of the isotope is registered. The logarithmic concentration curve reaches a rectilinear course within one minute and the curve is continued a few minutes longer. The blood pressure cuff is then inflated to a pressure which arrests isotope clearance (the clearance curve remains horizontal) and finally deflated 10 mm every two minutes until the isotope curve clears once again (Fig. 4).

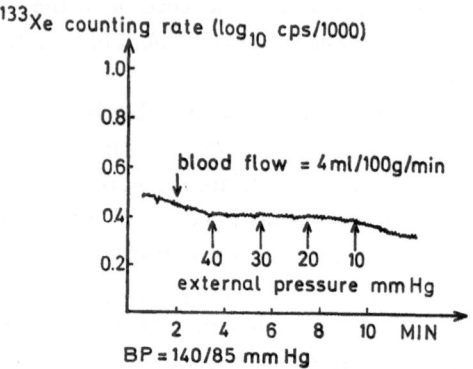

Fig. 4. A clearance curve obtained after intradermal injection of 0.1 ml histamin-^{133}Xe in saline solution in the dorsum of the foot. The patient had a peripheral gangrene due to arteriosclerotic occlusion of the arteries to the leg. The skin blood flow was calculated to be 4 ml/100 g . min, which is severely reduced (the average value in normal individuals is 16 ml/100 g . min). There is a pronounced distal hypotension as the counterpressure required to arrest the ^{133}Xe clearance is only 20 mm Hg (normally the distal blood pressure approximately equals the diastolic blood pressure).

Calculations: The maximum skin blood flow (SBF) can be determined by SBF = 100 · λ · ln(10) · D ml/100 g · min = 161 · D ml/100 g · min, where D is the steepest slope of the tangent to the logarithmic clearance curve, measured as that fraction of a decade which the tangent decreases in one minute.

The distal blood pressure (driving pressure) is taken as that external counter pressure in mm Hg which just arrests the ^{133}Xe clearance.

Results: Normal values: Skin blood flow: for this technique the maximum skin blood flow at the dorsum of the foot is 16.4 ml/100 g · min (SD = 5.9 ml/100 g ·min).

Distal blood pressure: the driving pressure of a vascular bed approximately equals the diastolic arterial blood pressure.

Clinical values: Skin blood flow: the maximal skin blood flow at the dorsum of the foot is severely reduced in patients with manifest or impending gangrene due to an occlusion of the main arteries to the leg. In the most pronounced cases the skin blood flow is nearly zero when the patient is tested in horizontal position (i.e the isotope clearance curve is a horizontal line).

Distal blood pressure: in patients with manifest or impending gangrene there is a pronounced low pressure area of the foot. The driving pressure is below 20-30 mm Hg.

Case 2. A 50 years old male with atherosclerotic arterial disease, who had previously had a mid-thig amputation of the right leg, developed gangrene of the 4th and 5th toes of his left foot. A further major amputation would have confined the patient permanently to his bed; thus in order to determine whether a conservative approach was feasible, blood pressure measurements were made after the injection of 133-Xenon histamine into the skin of the foot. On the medial side of the foot the local blood pressure was 70 mm Hg and on the lateral side, 15 mm Hg (fig. 5). Previous experience in the treatment of patients with severe peripheral arterial disease has shown that a pressure above 40 mm Hg is usually compatible with good healing. In the normal course of events the present patient's leg would have been amputated below the knee but in view of the relatively high pressure on the medial side of the foot, a local amputation was carried out. There was some sloughing in the wound but after removal, healing was satisfactory.

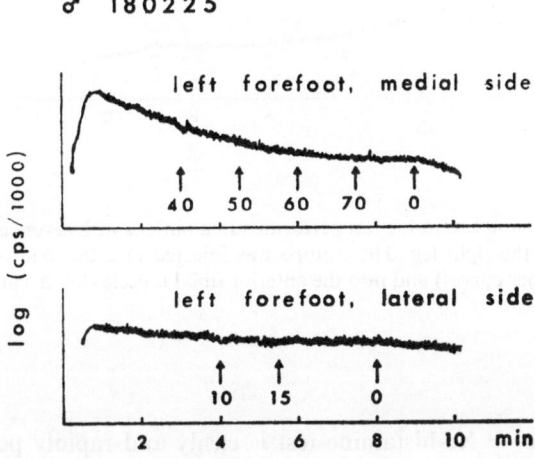

Fig. 5. The 133-Xenon histamine test performed in a patient with severe arterial occlusion of the arteries to the left leg. The isotope was injected intradermally at the medial and lateral sides of the left forefoot. (For further details, see text).

Case 3. A 65 years old man with atherosclerotic peripheral arterial disease had severe ischaemia of his right foot with rest pain. All peripheral pulses were absent below the femoral. It was decided that amputation was necessary and in order to determine the level of amputation, distal pressure and blood flow studies were carried out. Using the 133-Xenon histamine test, skin blood flow was measured on the dorsum of the foot (fig. 6). In the horizontal position and 'sitting up', the skin blood flow was zero. Only when the patient dangled his feet did a very slow clearance of the isotope occur, indicating severe ischaemia of the foot. Blood pressure in the anterior tibial muscle was found to be 30 mm Hg. This was thought too low a value to give satisfactory healing after a distal amputation and amputation above the knee was recommended.

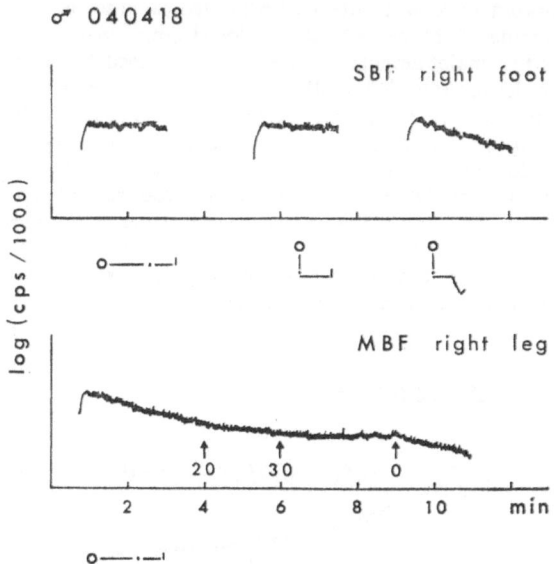

Fig. 6. The 133-Xenon histamine test performed in a patient with severe arterial occlusion of the arteries to the right leg. The isotope was injected into the skin of the dorsum of the right foot (upper curves) and into the anterior tibial muscle (lower curve). (For further details, see text).

Comments: The [133] Xe-histamine test is easily and rapidly performed. The entire test including calculations requires only 15-20 minutes and can be performed by a nurse or technician.

In special cases with occlusions of the arteries distal to the point of injection (some cases of Buerger's disease or diabetes), gangrene can be present in spite of the fact that the driving pressure and blood flow are normal or only slightly reduced at the dorsum of the foot. It is a little more difficult to diagnose such cases with the present technique, but the isotope-histamine solution can be injected more distally than the dorsum of the foot, e.g. in the skin at the base of the toes, the heel or the edge of the foot.

When a low-pressure area is verified at foot level it is often important to evaluate how proximal such an area is. By injecting 0.1 ml of the mixture of histamine and ^{133}Xe in saline into a distal muscle of the leg (usually m. tibialis anterior), the maximum blood flow in that area can be measured by following the clearance of the xenon radioactivity as described above. In normal man the maximum blood flow averages 34.7 ml/100 g·min (SD = 9.8 ml/100 g·min), and in the gangrene-prone distal vascular bed of patients with arterial occlusion it is reduced to an average of 7.3 ml/100 g·min (SD = 3.4 ml/100 g·min).

The distal blood pressure can also be measured in this area as that external counter pressure required to arrest the ^{133}Xe clearance when a blood pressure cuff is applied around the depot. Here too the driving pressure in normal man equals the diastolic blood pressure and is notably less in patients with severe arterial occlusion.

This test is not only used for diagnostic purposes. We can inject the xenon isotope into the skin or muscles at different levels in the leg or foot and thereby determine the distribution of the distal low pressure area – information of essential importance for the planning of amputations. Two examples illustrate this.

Clinical judgment in the planning and execution of amputation in peripheral arterial disease is of paramount importance. However, quantitative measurements of local blood pressure and blood flow can provide further information which can be invaluable in the management of these cases.

With the xenon method it is also easy to control the effect of a given treatment. In order to prove that a given treatment is of any value to the patient it must be demonstrated that the distal blood pressure and the distal blood flow have increased.

REFERENCES

1. Alpert, J., Garcia del Rio, H. & Lassen, N. A., Diagnostic use of radioactive xenon clearance and a standardized walking test in obliterative arterial disease of the legs. *Circulation* 34, 849-855 (1966).

2. Alpert, J., Larsen, O. A. & Lassen, N. A., Evaluation of arterial insufficiency of the legs. A comparison of arteriography and the ^{133}Xe walking test. *Cardiovasc. Res.* 2, 161-169 (1968).

3. Lassen, N. A., Lindbjerg, I. & Munck, O., Measurement of blood flow through skeletal muscle by intramuscular injection of Xenon-133. *Lancet* 1, 686-689 (1964).

4. Lindbjerg, I. F., Leg muscle blood-flow measured with [133]Xenon after ischaemia periods and after muscular exercise performed during ischaemia. *Clin. Sci.* 30, 399-408 (1966).

5. Larsen, O. A. & Lassen, N. A., Medical treatment of occlusive arterial disease of the legs. *Angiologica* 6, 288-301 (1966).

6. Lindbjerg, I. F., Measurement of muscle blood-flow with ^{133}Xe after histamine injection as a diagnostic method in peripheral arterial disease. *Scand. J. clin. Lab. Invest.* 17, 371-380 (1965).

7. Nilsen, R., Dahn, I., Lassen, N. A. & Westling, H., On the estimation of local effective perfusion pressure in patients with obliterative arterial disease by means of external compression over a Xenon-133 depot. *Scand. J. clin. Lab. Invest.* 19, suppl. 99, 29(1967).

PULSATILE BLOOD VELOCITY AND PRESSURE AND THE COMPUTER ANALYSIS OF CARDIOVASCULAR DATA

C. J. MILLS AND I. T. GABE

Blood pressure and blood velocity can now be measured simultaneously, with relative ease, at the time of cardiac catheterisation. The capacity to make such measurements in the arterial system presents problems in interpretation and analysis. In this brief account we shall describe, first the waveforms recorded in the arterial circulation interpreting some aspects of the changes in wave form that are seen; secondly we shall give an account of the use of a small digital computer to process some of the records.

ARTERIAL BLOOD FLOW AND PRESSURE WAVE FORMS

The device used to measure blood pressure and blood velocity is a catheter-tip electromagnetic velocity probe similar to that described previously (1). The size of the catheter is that of a No. 7F cardiac catheter, 2.3 mm o.d. It can be sterilized by autoclaving and is normally inserted percutaneously into an artery and advanced to the site where measurements are required.

Blood pressure and velocity wave forms in the systemic circulation are shown in figure 1. It will be observed that the waveform of pressure is quite different from that of velocity at most sites. The peak of velocity precedes the corresponding peak of pressure and there are periods during diastole when the blood velocity is close to zero. The difference in shape between the waveforms of pressure and velocity is due to the fact that the bed into which the flow is passing is not entirely resistive but contains elastic and inertial elements as well. Changes in the waveforms as the measuring site moves towards the periphery can be explained at least in part by the occurrence of reflections of pressure and velocity waves from the periphery. The system is complex and contains many separate reflecting sites. For the purpose of clarification it will be useful to consider a simple model system in which the essential features of reflection are exposed.

Consider first the propagation of a flow pulse along a simple lossless

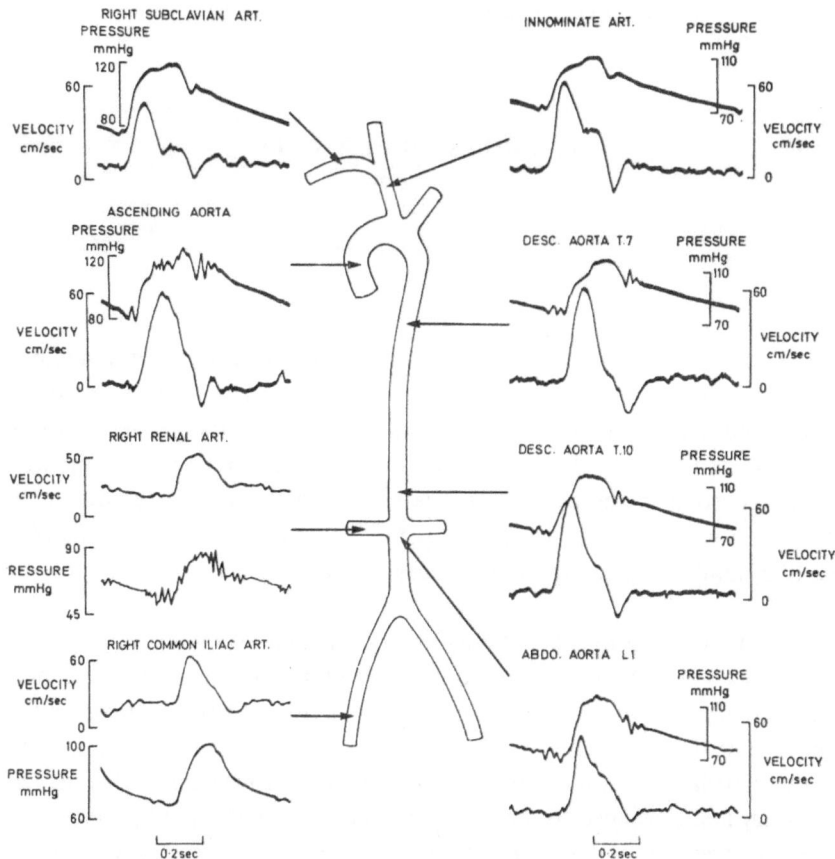

Fig. 1. Blood pressure and velocity waveforms recorded at points in the human systemic circulation. All the records were taken from one patient with the exception of traces from the right renal artery and right common iliac artery.

elastic tube containing a fluid. The system is shown in diagramatic form in figure 2. The tube is terminated in a complete obstruction at the point T so that no flow can pass at that point. Let us suppose that a forward flow wave has been created and is travelling from left to right along the tube. As it passes site 1 we may represent the forward flow wave as the shape F_1. The wave will continue to travel towards the obstruction and when it reaches the obstruction it may be represented as F_T. F_T will start some time after the beginning of F_1, the exact timing depending upon the distance travelled and the pulse wave velocity. Since no flow can pass the obstruction at T it follows that a backward wave B_T must be generated at the obstruction opposite in sign to F_T. The sum of F_T and B_T will be zero, since no flow is permitted at the obstruction. Once the backward wave, B_T, has been generated it will travel back along the tube, reaching site I after a delay and its shape at that point is represented in figure 2 as the wave form B_1. The actual flow pulse

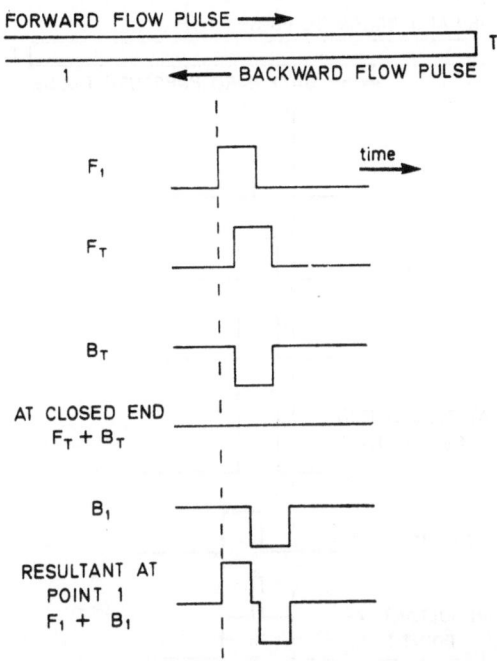

Fig. 2. Flow pulse propagation in a closed-end system. The upper part of this figure represents a long lossless, cylindrical elastic tube filled with fluid and terminated in a complete obstruction at the point T. Observations of flow are made at T and also at point I. See text.

that will be observed at site I is the sum of F_1 and B_1. Precise results and wave form will depend upon a number of factors; in the example shown in figure 2 a plateau is created in the middle of the wave form.

We consider now the results of a pressure pulse travelling in the same lossless fluid filled elastic tube terminated in a complete obstruction at T. The system and the waveforms produced are shown in figure 3. Let us suppose that we have created a forward pressure pulse and that the form of that pulse is as shown as F_1. At the site I. The pressure pulse will travel along the tube and by the time it reaches T it will have the form shown as F_T. No flow is permitted at the obstruction T and it follows, from the law of conservation of energy, that a backward pressure wave B_T must be generated at that point, similar in sign to F_T. The actual pressure at T will be the sum of F_T and B_T. The backward wave will pass from right to left and, as it passes site 1, it will have the form B_1. The resultant pressure at site 1 will be the sum of F_1 and B_1.

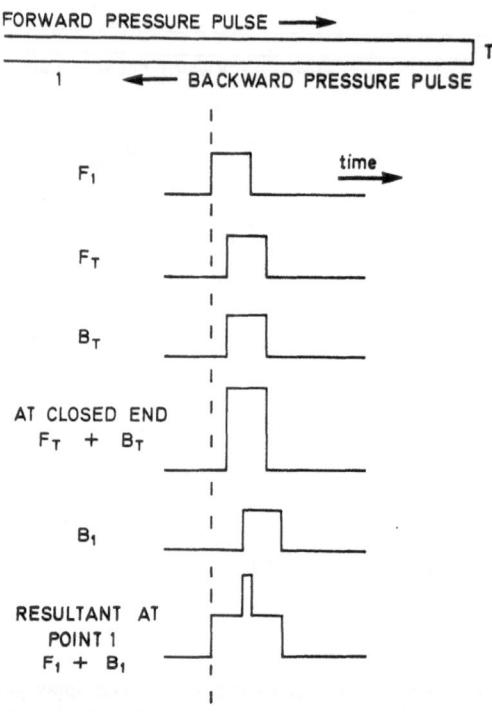

Fig. 3. Pressure pulse propagation in closed-end system. The upper part of this figure shows again a long, cylindrical elastic lossless tube containing fluid and terminated in a complete obstruction at the point T. Observations of pressure are made at T and also at point 1. See text.

Let us return now to figure 1. It will be seen that the narrower forward velocity pulse seen in the descending aorta, in comparison with the broader pulse in the ascending aorta, is compatible with flow reflections from at least a partially closed end. The plateau on the descending limb of the velocity waveform seen at L1 occurs later at T10 and later still at T7. The increasing delay is compatible with a forward wave interacting with a backward wave. Estimates of the timing are given in Mills, Gabe, Gault, Mason, Ross, Braunwald and Shillingford (2). In the innominate artery blood velocity pattern there is again a narrowing of the forward velocity pulse, followed by a plateau. Two other types of velocity pattern seen in the innominate artery are described in Mills et al. (2). It is likely that the changes seen in the later part of the velocity pulse in the innominate artery are the result of reflections coming from the descending aorta and passing into the innominate artery. Support for this hypothesis can be obtained by slowing the pulse wave velocity down in the descending aorta by means of the Valsalva manoeuvre. The plateau should then appear later in the cycle. The Valsalva manoeuvre slows the pulse wave velocity by reducing the transmural pressure and thus making the working arterial compliance larger. The result of a Valsalva manoeuvre on innominate artery blood velocity is shown in figure 4. Before the manoeuvre there was a plateau on the downslope of velocity. As the strain starts the plateau moves to points later in the cycle until a second forward wave appears during diastole. After release of the strain the initial blood velocity pattern returns.

The changes described here may seem to be of somewhat academic importance. Their relevance to present-day investigation is that they emphasize the importance of making central measurements of pressure and flow if cardiac performance is to be studied.

ANALYSIS OF PRESSURE AND VELOCITY WITH A DIGITAL COMPUTER

The ability to record blood pressure and velocity with ease results in the acquisition of large amounts of analogue data, and the processing of this data can pose formidable problems. We have used a digital computer to help in the analysis of the data and we shall now describe the main features of the system employed.

The digital computer used is the PDP-12. It has eight external analogue-to-digital conversion channels which enable records of pressure and velocity to be converted into digital form for storage on the two magnetic tape units which form an essential part of the computer. Once the data has been stored on the magnetic tape it can be displayed on an oscilloscope screen so that the validity of the records can be checked. The main language in which we have written the programmes is Fortran. Because the computer is a small one it was necessary to divide the programme up into a series of 'chapters', each of which is stored on one of the magnetic tape units. The sequence of chapters required for a three channel version, capable of dealing with aortic pressure, ventricular pressure and aortic flow is shown in figure 5. The chapters are called automatically into use as the need arises. Several of the chapters contain machine language programmes for analogue to digital conversion and for display of variables on the oscilloscope screen. The system has been written in such a way that the operator must interact with the

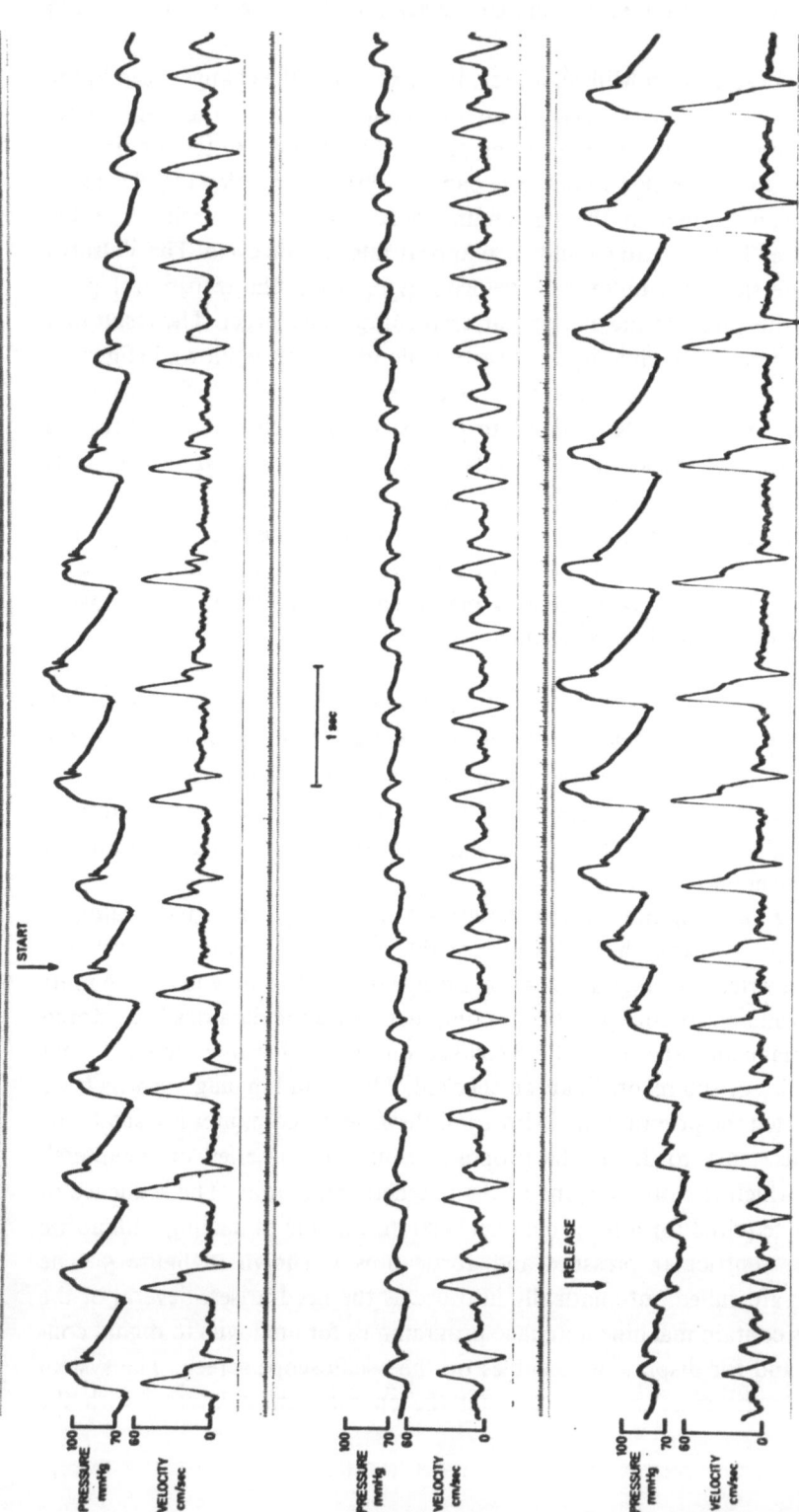

Fig. 4. A continuous record of pressure and blood velocity in the innominate artery of a patient during a Valsalva manoeuvre. Observe the changes in the velocity pattern during the strain. There were reasons for believing that part of the change in waveform is the result of reflections from the descending aorta entering the innominate artery later during the strain than before or afterwards. During a Valsalva manoeuvre pulse wave velocity will be decreased

SEQUENCE OF CHAPTERS FOR FORTRAN-LINC SYSTEM

3-CHANNEL VERSION

AORTIC PRESSURE, VENTRICULAR PRESSURE AND AORTIC FLOW

CHAPTER 1 – CALIBRATION A/D
CHAPTER 2 – CALIBRATION CONT. PRINT CALIBRATION CONSTANTS
CHAPTER 3 – A/D, STORE DATA ON TAPE AND DISPLAY
CHAPTER 4 – COMPUTE BASIC HAEMODYNAMIC VALUES
CHAPTER 5 – COMPUTE BASIC HAEMODYNAMIC VALUES – CONT.
CHAPTER 6 – PRINT BASIC HAEMODYNAMIC VALUES
CHAPTER 7 – COMPUTE BEAT-TO-BEAT VALUES
CHAPTER 8 – COMPUTE BEAT-TO-BEAT VALUES – CONT.
CHAPTER 9 – PRINT BEAT-TO-BEAT VALUES
CHAPTER 10 – REDISPLAY DATA
CHAPTER 11 – COMPUTE VENTRICULAR CHARACTERISTICS
CHAPTER 12 – PREPARE TO FLOAT
CHAPTER 13 – FLOAT, CUT, STACK AND AVERAGE
CHAPTER 14 – FOURIER ANALYSIS + CALIBRATION + CORRECTION
CHAPTER 15 – POLAR CONVERSION
CHAPTER 16 – COMPUTE VASCULAR IMPEDANCE
CHAPTER 17 – PRINT RESULTS AND PLOT IMPEDANCE

Fig. 5. The list of programmes (each termed a 'chapter') written to analyse aortic pressure, ventricular pressure and aortic flow on a PDP-12 computer.

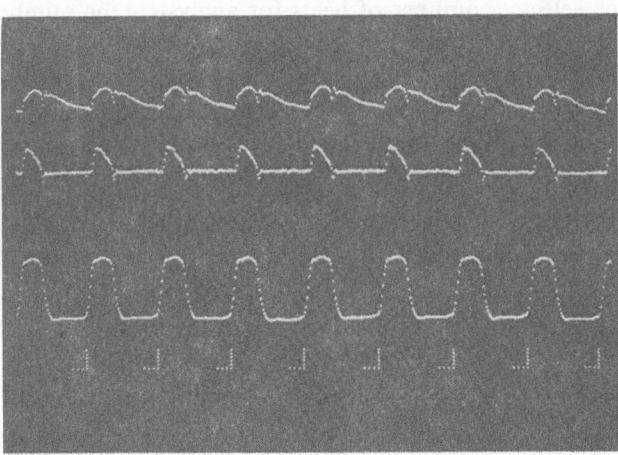

Fig. 6. An example of the display of aortic pressure, aortic velocity and left ventricular pressure waveforms after analogue-to-digital conversion.

computer through the teletype and select and judge data as it passes through the system. Thus, for example, after analogue-to-digital conversion the data seen on the screen may be similar to that shown in figure 6. The traces from above downwards are of aortic pressure, aortic velocity and left ventricular pressure. Further beats can be brought on to the screen by touching a switch, the total number of beats capable of being displayed in this way being 128. If there are artefacts on the records these can be quickly identified and analogue-to-digital conversion can be restarted.

The output of one of the main programmes used is shown in figure 7. The teletype prints the question 'No. of beats for basic P, V and LV'. The

```
→ NO. OF BEATS FOR BASIC P,V & LV:10
  H.R.=  95.5 ; S.E.=  0.13

       MAX -- SE    MIN -- SE     AV -- SE    DYDT - SEDY   TDY - SETDY
  P   135.4  0.6   93.1  0.3   114.2  0.4    710   46.2    68.0  19.1
  V   190.4  1.3  -58.4  1.8    32.5  0.4   4591   153     62.0   2.0
  LV  136.8  0.5   17.2  1.0    55.3  0.7   2051   18.0   215.0  94.2

  TRUE ZERO-CAL ZERO =-355.3
  FLOW=(  1.948   X AREA) L/MIN
  S.V.=( 20.388   X AREA) ML
  P.R.=  4690

→ EXIT?0
```

Fig. 7. An example of the output after computation of a set of programmes designed to compute average values of a set of beats. In this example ten beats have been analysed.

operator then selects a number of beats for analysis – the number must be less than 128 – and in the example chosen ten beats have been analysed. The average heart rate is then calculated as 95.5 beats per minute with a standard error of the mean over the ten beats of 0.13. The digitalised data over the ten beats is then examined and about one minute later the main information in figure 7 is typed out. It will be seen that pressure velocity and left ventricular pressure information is dealt with and that, for example, the maximum that the systolic pressure averaged over the ten beats is 135.4 mm Hg with a standard error of .6, that the peak flow is 190.4 ml/sec. (calibration has been carried out in terms of flow in this instance, not velocity), with a standard error of 1.3 and that the systolic left ventricular pressure was 136.8 mm Hg with a standard error of .5. Similarly, it is possible to have information on the average diastolic pressure, left ventricular end-diastolic pressure, mean pressures and rates of change of pressure. In this way it is possible to obtain representative average values over any number of beats up to 128 and to obtain with ease statistical information about important levels. At the end of

the print-out the word 'exit' is typed and this gives the operator the opportunity of leaving this programme and returning to the analogue-to-digital
programme so that further records can be analysed. Thus it is possible to
obtain basic haemodynamic information in digital form every two to three
minutes during a procedure. Normally we obtain information by recording
on an analogue tape recorder and analyse it later; however it is possible to
operate the computer during an actual investigation.

There are occasions when it is desirable to obtain detailed information on
a series of beats. Thus, for example, figure 8 shows the result of inflating a

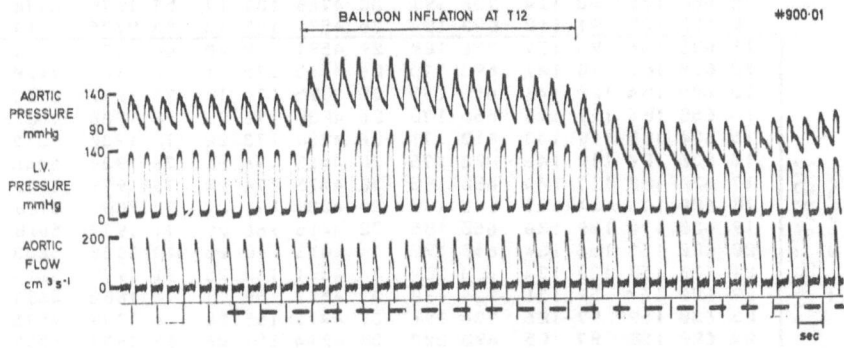

Fig. 8. A record of aortic pressure, left ventricular pressure and aortic flow before, during
and after inflation of a balloon in the descending aorta at the level T-12.

balloon in the descending aorta at the level T12. There was a rise in aortic
pressure and left ventricular pressure and a fall in peak aortic velocity.
Analysis of this record on a beat-to-beat basis is possible and the results of
such a process is shown in figure 9. Forty beats have been analysed. It will
be seen that the balloon inflation extends from after beat 10 to after beat 27.
Inevitably this process takes longer than the averaging programme, largely
because of the greater time required for typing the results.

The final set of programmes is concerned with taking pressure and velocity information, calculating the Fourier harmonics and computing the
vascular impedance of the bed concerned. An example of a print-out of this
kind of information is shown in figure 10. Eight beats have been chosen for a
particular form of averaging appropriate to the problem. The vascular impedance is calculated and printed in modulus and phase angle form and is
shown beneath the letter Z on the right of the figure. It is possible to plot the
vascular impedance on an XY plotter so that manual graphing of the results
is not necessary.

C. J. MILLS AND I. T. GABE

→ NO. OF BEATS FOR BEAT TO BEAT: 40

H.R.= 95.8 ; S.E.= 0.12

	T	SP	DP	MP	D	SV	MV	D	SLV	EDP	MLV	D	PR
0													
1	630	135	93	114	736	196	32	4944	136	25	54	2075	4751
2	630	133	93	112	736	191	33	4591	135	13	52	2027	4554
3	630	138	93	116	736	191	35	4944	138	17	57	2075	4450
4	630	137	95	115	779	189	34	4944	138	17	56	2075	4576
5	620	135	93	114	743	192	35	3708	137	16	56	1930	4340
6	630	134	94	113	736	196	31	4768	136	14	53	2075	4781
7	630	137	93	116	736	187	33	3708	138	19	58	2123	4730
8	630	138	93	115	779	187	30	4944	138	19	57	2075	5142
9	620	135	93	114	736	191	32	4768	137	17	57	1979	4770
10	630	132	91	112	823	184	30	4591	135	13	53	2075	4917
11	630	168	96	137	736	189	29	4591	160	20	64	2075	6377
12	630	183	118	147	693	170	26	4415	175	21	72	2123	7420
13	600	184	122	148	650	175	30	3885	176	18	75	1979	6703
14	650	184	119	146	650	170	26	4238	176	21	72	1930	7586
15	630	180	118	143	650	171	26	4238	173	22	72	1930	7313
16	630	184	119	146	693	175	30	4415	176	25	76	1930	6446
17	630	180	117	144	650	182	32	4415	174	24	76	1979	6039
18	620	177	114	141	693	180	30	4238	171	24	75	1882	6188
19	630	172	109	136	650	185	32	4415	166	22	71	1979	5698
20	620	165	106	134	650	192	34	4415	160	25	70	1930	5243
21	630	168	107	134	693	189	34	4591	162	25	71	1979	5214
22	620	164	59	131	736	192	37	4591	159	8	70	1882	4687
23	630	159	99	126	736	196	37	4415	155	22	66	1979	4575
24	620	158	97	125	693	203	38	4944	154	26	67	1979	4382
25	630	157	98	124	736	203	38	5121	153	26	68	1930	4356
26	620	153	94	121	779	210	40	4944	151	25	67	1930	4075
27	620	145	83	113	779	212	44	5121	144	21	62	1882	3436
28	630	132	74	102	736	219	44	5121	134	24	59	1834	3106
29	620	122	54	88	866	228	44	5474	126	22	56	1737	2661
30	620	104	46	73	1039	244	50	6004	115	17	48	1786	1955
31	620	96	45	67	1126	240	46	6357	108	15	42	1834	1939
32	630	97	43	67	1213	247	47	6180	109	17	44	1882	1895
33	620	96	43	66	1126	245	49	6004	107	15	42	1882	1789
34	620	95	41	65	1256	245	45	6357	106	12	39	1930	1904
35	630	92	41	63	1256	242	42	6180	103	6	34	1930	1986
36	630	95	42	67	1169	240	41	6180	105	9	37	1979	2165
37	630	95	44	68	1256	237	39	6534	102	10	35	1882	2313
38	620	96	49	69	1126	233	39	6180	103	7	34	1979	2344
39	630	95	48	71	1126	235	40	6004	102	10	35	1930	2354
40	620	99	54	76	1126	237	38	6180	107	8	37	2027	2677

BALLOON INFLATION (rows 11–27)

Fig. 9. Results of analysing forty beats shown in analogue form in Fig. 8. The letters at the top of the column signify, in order, the period of each beat in milliseconds, systolic pressure, diastolic pressure, mean pressure, maximum rate of change of aortic pressure, systolic velocity, mean velocity, acceleration, systolic left ventricular pressure, end-diastolic pressure, mean left ventricular pressure, maximum rate of change of left ventricular pressure and peripheral resistance.

The labour involved in programming the digital computer has been considerable. It has taken the two of us more than a year to bring it to the present stage. Certainly, data processing is now comparatively simple and rapid, and problems can be now approached that previously seemed to be too time consuming.

```
--> NO OF R-R INTERVALS FOR STACK:8        ****

    AV. NO. OF SAMPLES/BEAT: 62.875 ;    63 ;S.D.= .3536
    AV. HT. RATE FREQ. 1.5905 PER SEC.
--> NO. HARMONICS REQD.:8
    TRUE ZERO - CAL. ZERO:-355.3


    CODE NO=  900.01  TIME=15.14
         -F-      ---P---        ---V---        ---Z---
    0    0.00  114.431    0.0   32.428    0.0   4704    0.0    0
    1    1.59   15.812  118.8   66.282   59.1    318  -59.7    1
    2    3.18    6.571  133.7   51.895  122.5    169  -11.2    2
    3    4.77    4.529 -170.2   31.110 -176.1    194   -6.0    3
    4    6.36    1.280 -133.5   10.727 -145.6    159  -12.2    4
    5    7.95    1.093  157.8   10.439 -171.6    140   30.6    5
    6    9.54    1.734 -171.1   11.228 -119.9    206   51.2    6
    7   11.13    1.472  -99.8    8.262  -54.2    238   45.6    7
    8   12.72    0.024 -129.9    0.821  -83.6     38   46.3    8

--> PLOT OPTION:2 NO HARMONICS:7  HZCAL=10  MODCAL=2000
```

Fig. 10. The result of Fourier analysis of pressure and velocity waveforms, averaged over eight beats, is shown in the lower part of this figure. The Fourier components are shown in modulus and phase angle form and the vascular impedance is shown on the right beneath the letter Z.

REFERENCES

1. Mills, C. J. & Shillingford, J. P., A catheter tip electromagnetic velocity probe and its evaluation. *Cardiovasc. Res.* 1, 263-273 (1967).

2. Mills C. J., Gabe, I. T., Gault, J. H., Mason, D. T., Ross, J. Jr., Braunwald, E. & Shillingford, J. P., Pressure-flow relationships and vascular impedance in man. *Cardiovasc. Res.* 4, 405-417 (1970).

DISCUSSION

Audience: I would like to ask if varicose veins have any influence on the measurement of the wash-out of xenon from the muscle.

Larsen: Using the local isotope clearance principle, Xenon-133 is injected into the muscle tissue and is then removed by the blood flow in the muscle capillaries. Theoretically, an increase in the pressure at the venous end of the capillary could lead to a decrease in the pressure gradient over the capillary and the flow should therefore decrease. During routine use of the Xenon Walking Test we have not observed any decrease in blood flow during walking in patients with varicose veins, but to my knowledge no systematic investigation of this problem has been carried out.

Audience: You started your talk by saying you used a standardized treadmill test. Can you tell exactly how you standardized that test?

Larsen: With the Xenon-133 standardized walking test we measure the muscle blood flow at the site and at the moment the patient develops ischaemic pain. After injection of the isotope the subject stands motionless on the treadmill for 3 to 5 minutes, while the resting muscle clearance is measured. Thereafter the patient walks until fatigue and pain in the leg stop him. The speed of the treadmill is normally 4.5 km/h. The elevation of the treadmill is either 8% or 16% and patients are tested using the steepest grade on which they can walk for about 2 minutes. The patient should walk as normally as possible with a step of 70 cm and wear ordinary low-heeled walking shoes. After the walking test the patient stands motionless until the hyperemic phase in the leg muscles has passed. The walking test can be reproduced fairly reasonably, with a coefficient of variation of about 8% in repeated testing of patients with maximum walking distances of about 2 minutes.

Audience: Don't you think that the blood flow is partly dependant on the load you apply? I should think it was.

Larsen: I think so too, and therefore we try to apply a maximum or rather submaximum load.

Audience: In which way does training affect the results?

Larsen: Patients with a good clinical result following walking training show flow changes which, with respect to all curve parameters analyzed, change in the direction of a normalization. We observe after training an increase in maximum blood flow during and after walking, a decrease in the time between cessation of walking and re-establishment of resting blood flow and a decrease in the remaining hyperemia after walking. Our interpretation of these results and results from other studies is that the effect of training in patients with chronic intermittent claudication is not due to a more effective collateral circulation, but to more efficient enzymatic systems in the muscle tissue. Both animal and human studies have shown that muscle tissue in trained subjects contains more and bigger mitochondria, which means that more oxygen can be extracted from the same amount of blood. Furthermore we think that the amount of blood in the proximal muscles of the leg is less in the trained patients than in the untrained. This means that more blood will be available to the distal muscles in the leg.

Audience: Do you think that there is much oxygen left to take by training? The oxygen pressure is usually very low in the saphenous veins especially during maximum work.

Larsen: It has been shown by Swedish investigators that the oxygen saturation and lactate concentration measured in the femoral vein during maximum work are lower in trained than in untrained subjects. This suggests that the muscle tissue in trained patients has more efficient enzymatic systems.

Audience: Do you agree that the disappearance of xenon in muscles is mulitexponential? If so, what is the cause or what are the origins of the exponents?

Larsen: It is correct that the muscle blood flow curve is multi-exponential, but this will not invalidate the routine tests I have described. The main reason for the multi-exponential appearance is that when xenon leaves the muscle tissue it can diffuse out through the walls of the small veins; it is then fixated in the fatty tissue and from there is cleared very slowly.

Sayers: I do not think there is any doubt that in the clearance curves diffusion processes occur which cannot really be described as a single exponential function. However, it nearly always turns out that the approximation by one exponential is indeed fair enough. The only circumstances known to me where it might be worth making a distinction between a single exponential and a distributed system is curiously enough in measurements of cardiac output. There I think that the approximation of a decay curve of an indicator is perhaps improved slightly by recognizing the nature of the underlying diffusion process. When an indicator is injected into the system, it not only diffuses outwards from the site of injection (which is a symmetrical process in a perfectly static fluid bed), but it of course also drifts because of the blood flow so that with diffusion there is also drift. If you look further down the system you can in fact see that the way in which the indicator concentration rises and then falls is rather better described by solving the particular equation arising from such a model.

Gabe: Could I ask a question about whether estimates of cardiac output are better when you take the factors that you have mentioned into consideration. Has that been done?

Sayers: Yes, that has been done. It only matters when it is very difficult to actually identify from the indicator dilution curve where the negative exponential starts and finishes. Under normal conditions the exponential approximation is quite a good one.

Sheffield: I was fascinated by the probe that Dr. Mills and Dr. Gabe described a while ago and I would like to enquire about the possible uses they have planned for it. Could it for example have its output modified by a computer to give an estimation of cardiac output?

Mills: If you know the size of the vessel, certainly one can change the calibration into terms of flow. The velocity profile in the ascending aorta is relatively flat and therefore the position of the probe is not that important.

Audience: Could you use your probe in different parts of the circulation? What parts would be the most important for intensive care or postsurgical care for example?

Gabe: We ourselves have not really been much concerned with intensive care. We are mostly concerned with intensive investigation over quite short periods of time and the computer program which you saw is intended for short term experiments. We did not leave the catheter in for very long; I think the maximum time in man is something like 6 hours. I do not think anybody really knows what is best measured in terms of intensive care.

CHAPTER 4

CARDIAC RHYTHM

COMPUTER DETECTION AND ANALYSIS OF VENTRICULAR ECTOPIC RHYTHMS

J. M. NEILSON AND C. W. VELLANI

INTRODUCTION

Over the past three years we have been studying the patterns of ventricular arrhythmias in the electrocardiograms of 200 patients with acute myocardial infarction in the Coronary Care Unit of the Royal Infirmary, Edinburgh. The purpose of this study is to establish the natural history of ventricular ectopic beats after myocardial infarction and to determine whether coupling intervals of ectopic complexes in large samples of the ECG could give clues to the mechanisms of production. We report here our methods of data collection and analysis and the interpretation of some of our results.

METHODS

The bipolar chest lead electrocardiogram displayed for monitoring in the coronary care unit was recorded on magnetic tape continuously for 24-72 hours from the time of admission. The tape recording system used has been specially developed in the Department of Medical Physics. It records up to three ECG signals simultaneously using wide deviation (IRIG) frequency modulation recording at a record tape speed of 38 cm per minute. Standard 540 metre reels of tape allow twenty four hours of recording per reel. The tapes may be replayed at the original recording speed, or at 38 cm per second (sixty times faster) for high speed analysis. The bandwidth of the system is DC to 45 Hz (3 dB down). Electronic flutter compensation ensures that the overall peak to peak noise level introduced by the tape system is 40 dB down relative to full scale modulation. This means that the quality of the reproduced ECG signal is such that in many cases the resulting record is indistinguishable from the original.

In the high speed replay mode each twenty four hour tape is reviewed visually several times in the course of analysis. Using a suitable long persistence oscilloscope display, twenty four hours of ECG can be viewed in as many minutes and yet discrete events, even a solitary ventricular ectopic complex can be observed without difficulty. By slowing down to real time replay, events of particular interest can be recorded on standard ECG chart paper for detailed study.

Early in our work it was clear that such visual methods of analysis of the ECG signal are totally inadequate to deal with the very large amounts of data contained in the record for each patient, some of whom can produce well over ten thousand ventricular ectopic complexes in each twenty four hours. To handle this data effectively a special purpose analogue/hybrid electronic computer* has been developed to operate directly on the ECG signal during high speed replay detecting and timing the occurrence of individual ventricular ectopic complexes.

For the reasons that there is considerable variation in morphology of 'normal' QRS complexes seen in coronary care electrocardiograms and even greater variation of ventricular ectopic complexes and, not least, the poor signal to noise ratio in such monitoring signals, the computer has been designed to operate in a self adaptive mode. Recognition of ventricular ectopic complexes is based on the difference in morphology which they show in relation to the 'prevailing' QRS complex.

A block diagram of the computer is shown in figure 1A. The incoming ECG signal is processed in the trigger section where the QRS wave of each ECG complex is detected by filtering, differentiating and rectifying the signal. The background noise produced by P and T waves, muscle potentials, etc., is separately measured and used to control the level of an automatic threshold with which the processed signal is compared. Any QRS wave producing an output which is significantly above the level of noise prevailing at that time will be detected and used to generate a master trigger pulse controlling further operations on that complex.

The master trigger pulse occurs just before the QRS wave which generated it emerges from the solid state analogue delay line and enters the shape comparison section. In this section, under the control of the master trigger pulse, each QRS wave is sampled repeatedly for two hundred milliseconds starting in the PR segment and ending in the ST segment. One of the samples in the PR segment is used to establish the base-line level of the incoming waveform and, because the set of samples is locked in time relative to the arrival of the QRS wave, the samples so obtained for each QRS wave describe it within a 'reference frame' fixed relative to the wave in both time and voltage.

When a new electrocardiogram is first applied to the computer the oper-

---

* U.K. and overseas patents pending.

ator presses a 'Learn' switch during the passage of a QRS wave which he wishes the machine to accept as 'normal' for that particular patient. This causes the set of samples for that QRS wave to be transferred into the memory section of the machine where it is stored in analogue sample/hold stages. Thereafter, the samples acquired for every succeeding QRS wave are compar-

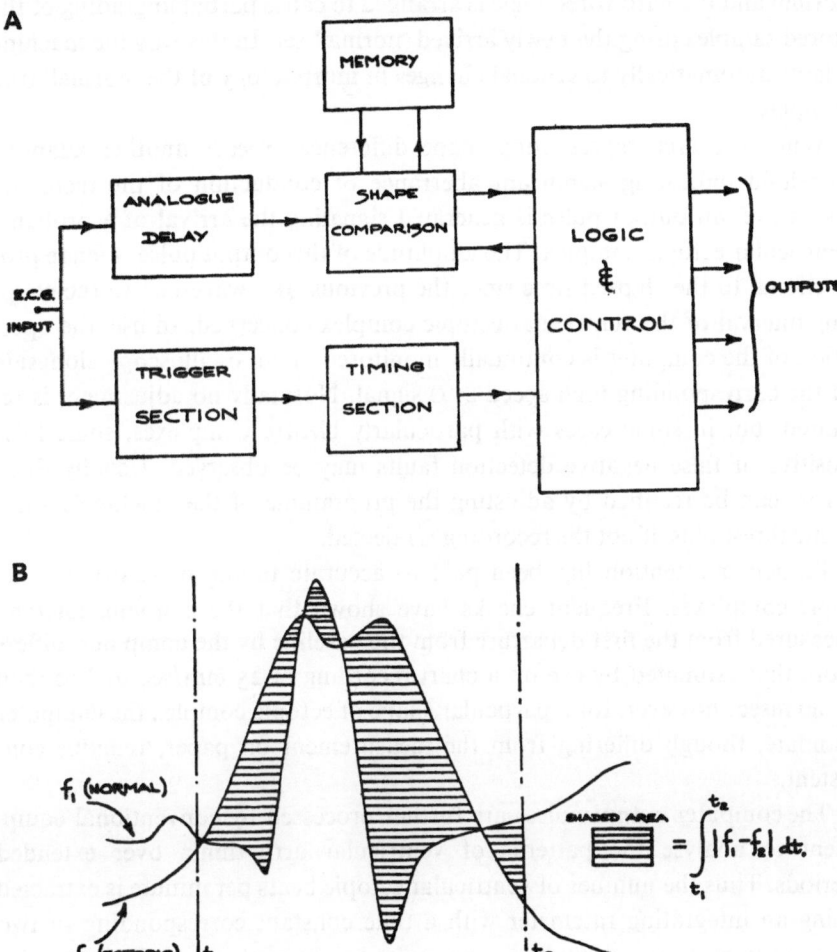

Fig. I. Computer detection of ventricular ectopic complexes.

ed with the 'normal' set in the memory. As each QRS wave is sampled in the same frame of reference, the samples are used to calculate the area not common to both the 'normal' QRS wave (f_1 figure 1b) and the QRS wave currently under examination (f_2) when the two waves are effectively superimposed. The area so calculated (shaded in figure 1b) is a measure of the difference in shape between the complex being examined and the stored 'normal' complex.

When this area is small in relation to that of the 'normal' QRS wave, signifying that the incoming QRS wave is a 'good fit', the complex is regarded as normal and the hard wired logic is arranged to cause partial upgrading of the stored samples using the newly arrived 'normal' set. In this way the machine adapts automatically to gradual changes in morphology of the 'normal' QRS complex.

When the area representing shape difference exceeds another adaptive threshold indicating significant aberrance of conduction of the incoming QRS wave, an output pulse is generated signaling the arrival of a probable ventricular ectopic complex. The amplitude of this output pulse is made proportional to the elapsed time since the previous QRS wave i.e., to the coupling interval of the ventricular ectopic complex concerned. In use, the operation of the computer is continually monitored on an oscilloscope alongside of the corresponding high speed ECG signal. Normally no adjustment is required, but in some cases with particularly bizarre complexes, some false positive or false negative detection faults may be observed. Usually these errors can be rectified by adjusting the programme of the machine's automatic thresholds, if not the recording is rejected.

Particular attention has been paid to accurate timing of ventricular ectopic complexes. Frequent checks have shown that the coupling interval, measured from the first departure from the baseline by the computer, differs from that estimated by eye on a chart recording at 25 mm/sec by less than ± 40 msec; however, for a particular shape of ectopic complex the computer estimate, though differing from the measurement on paper, remains consistent.

The computer output pulses are further processed by conventional equipment to analyse the patterns of ventricular arrhythmia over extended periods. Thus the number of ventricular ectopic beats per minute is extracted using an integrating ratemeter with a time constant corresponding to two minutes in real time. A multichannel pulse height analyser reads the amplitudes of the computer output pulses and plots histograms of the distribution of ectopic complexes in the cardiac cycle. Intervals between computer output pulses are measured separately by an analogue timer; its output, also in the form of pulses varying in amplitude proportional to the intervals, is similarly examined in histogram form using the pulse height analyser.

RESULTS

In the coronary care unit the usual finding is that ventricular ectopic beats are few and appear sporadically but there is often a period of an hour or less when the number of ectopic beats exceeds 5/min. On the other hand ectopic activity may be sustained decreasing gradually or may occur intermittently over many hours, each paroxysm terminating spontaneously (Fig. 2).

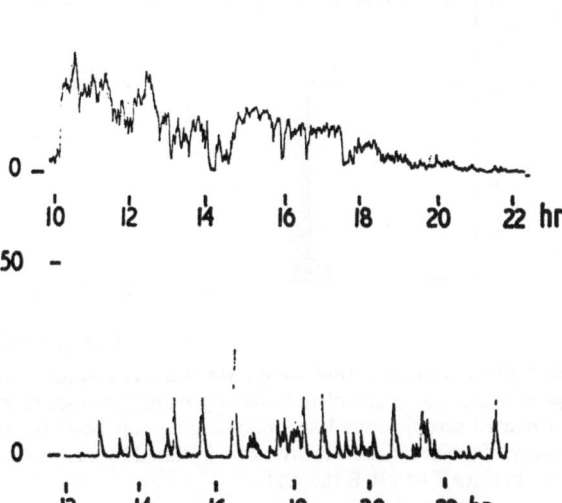

Fig. 2. Trend of numbers of ventricular ectopic beats appearing per minute in two patients with acute myocardial infarction.

Paroxysmal ectopic appearance makes assessment of the efficacy of antiarrhythmic therapy very difficult unless the trend can be clearly established before the drug is given. Short runs of consecutive ventricular beats usually lasting less than 30 secs occur in most patients.

There are many patterns of ectopic distribution in the cardiac cycle some of which have distinctive features. A characteristic but uncommon finding is the ectopic complex which appears early after the end of the T wave of the preceding complex and is fixed in this position whenever it appears (Fig. 3). Noteworthy of this type of beat is the fact that it is usually single but when a pair of beats appear, the coupling interval of the second ectopic to the first is shorter than the first to the sinus complex so that the second ectopic appears on the downstroke or apex of the T wave of the first. The 'R or T' phenomenon is more often of this kind than of the type in which the ectopic interrupts the T wave of a sinus beat. When the sequence described progresses to consecutive 'R or T' complexes, the ventricular rate is invariably greater than 200/min (Fig. 3).

A pattern which is uncommon in our experience is that in which the ectopic beats appear late in diastole and there is evidence that they are due to

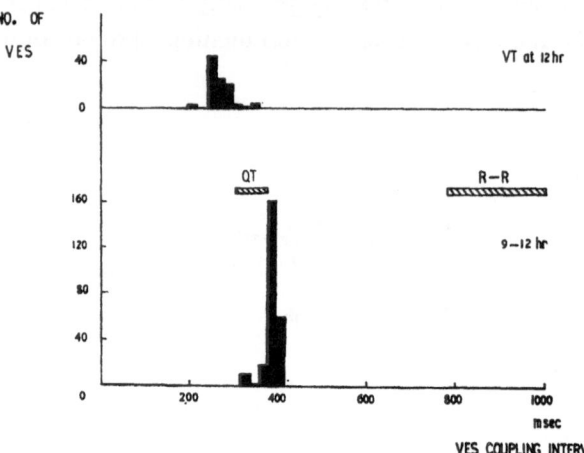

Fig. 3. Distribution of ventricular ectopic complexes at the end of the T wave. Coupling is fixed with a range of 60msec. A group of 10 beats at 320 and 340 msec represents the coupling interval of a pair of ectopic complexes following a sinus beat; the upper histogram shows the periodicity of the ventricular tachycardia initiated by such a sequence. The bars show the variations in sinus T and R-R intervals.

an escape mechanism. Figure 4 shows two distributions of ectopic beats

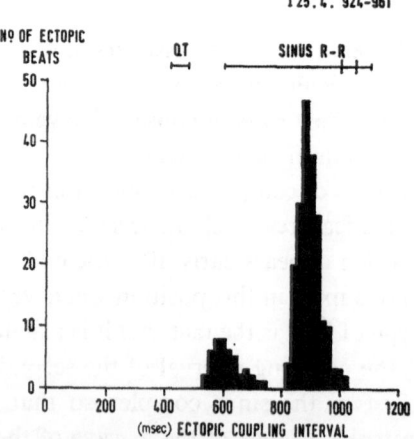

Fig. 4. Histogram of the distribution of two morphologically distinct ventricular ectopic beats appearing in a period of 50 minutes (See text). The cross bars on the range of sinus R-R intervals indicate peak frequency of these intervals.

representing morphologically distinct complexes which appeared in a 50 minute period during which the sinus period varied considerably but had a peak frequency between 1040 and 1100 msec. The ectopic distribution around 880 msec is the one under discussion; within this group two 7 minute samples with different prevailing sinus periods are shown in figure 5.

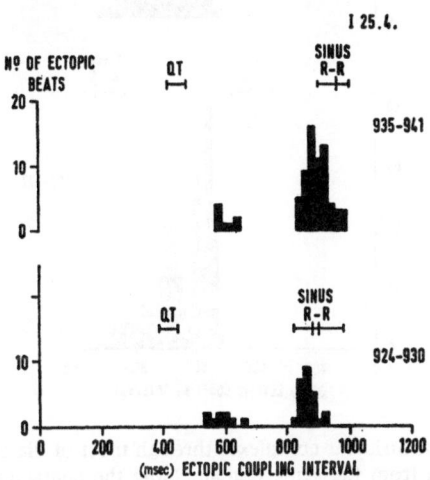

Fig. 5. Ectopic distribution in 2 seven minute periods within the sample shown in figure 4.

The shorter sinus period is associated with reduced numbers of ectopic beats sparing only that part of the group which has coupling intervals shorter than the prevailing sinus period. Appearance of these beats is dependent upon a sufficiently long sinus period and the ectopic pacemaker may be said to lack 'entrance block' (1).

Distribution of ectopic beats through most of diastole is the usual finding; there is however a tendency for the complexes to appear in one or more favourite positions which vary from time to time (Fig. 6). We believe that the distribution is due to ventricular parasystole, the ectopic pacemaker being 'protected' (1) from sinus conducted beats. Evidence for this is twofold. First-ly the numbers of ectopic beats do not decrease as a result of increasing sinus sinus rate. Secondly the ectopic coupling interval distribution is altered when the sinus period changes (Fig. 7a) while the pattern of intervals between ectopic beats shows little change (Fig. 7b). If the ectopic beats were fixed in time to the preceding sinus beats, the intervals between ectopic complexes would be expected to change with the sinus period. There may be several reasons for favourite coupling intervals; however the variable positions of

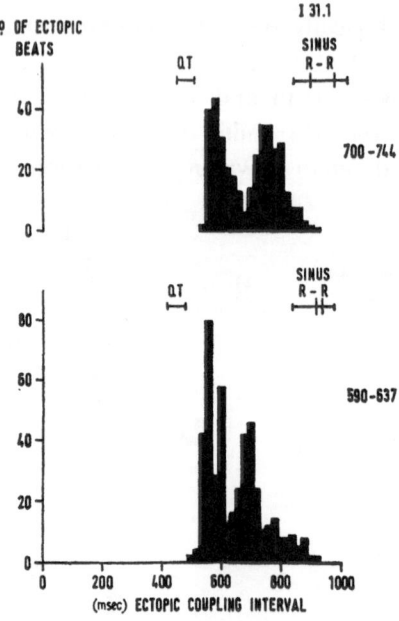

Fig. 6. Distribution of ventricular complexes through most of diastole in 2 samples each of 45 minutes duration from the same patient. Note the characteristic peaks and their variable positions in the two histograms.

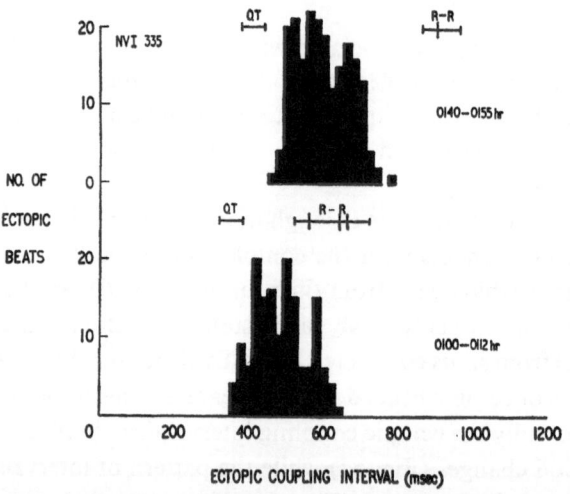

Fig. 7a and 7b. The distribution of ventricular ectopic beats changes with sinus rate while the intervals between ectopic beats and the number of beats appearing per minute tend to remain constant suggesting a mechanism of ectopic production which is independent of sinus rhythm.

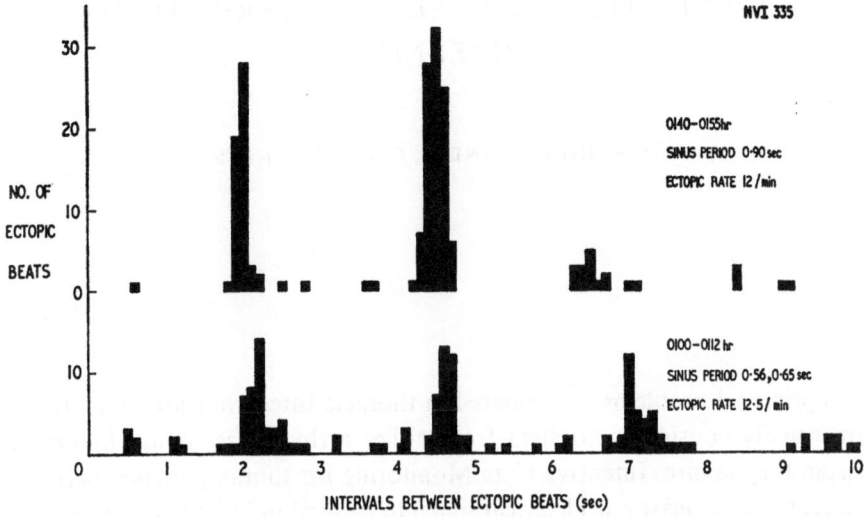

Fig. 7b.

the peaks in our coupling interval histograms suggest that a tendency for the ectopic pacemaker rate to synchronise with the sinus may be the usual method whereby ectopics appear to be fixed in a particular part of diastole.

The combination of changing ectopic coupling intervals with change in sinus rate together with constant inter-ectopic intervals strongly suggests an independent rhythm influenced, though seldom wholly captured, by sinus rhythm.

REFERENCES

1. Stock, J. P. P., *Diagnosis and treatment of cardiac arrhythmias*. p. 73. London 1970.

FIRST STEPS IN REAL-TIME ARRHYTHMIA SCREENING

M. R. HOARE AND A. C. ARNTZENIUS

The principal problems encountered in thoracic Intensive Care Units (ICU) are usually considered to stem from either arrhythmias, pump failure or respiratory failure. Intensive Care Monitoring for thorax patients therefore incorporates at least one electrical signal to be used in identifying or predicting such occurrences. Various basic systems are in current use to monitor these signals ranging from a nurse with a chart recorder via simple analogue circuits and dedicated analogue or digital computers to complex information systems based on large digital computers or networks. Each basic system has different clinical or economic justifications for its use. All have in common that they accept one or more electrical signals (electrocardiogram, pressure wave) as input and act as data-concentrators providing the clinician with a particular selection from, and evaluation of, their input information.

Multiple ICU's for coronary, respiratory and post-operative patients were set up at the Thorax Centre of the Medische Faculteit Rotterdam. These units were designed to be computer-aided using a small central digital computer (a DEC PDP-9) in an attempt to provide monitoring flexibility without great cost. The electrical signals available from each unit would not necessarily be the same and each group of patients would certainly differ in their monitoring needs. Agreement was reached, however, that all patients in all units (a total of 20 patients) might require continuous monitoring of their ECG's. No computer system available in 1969 would or could handle 20 beds with a single computer even had ECG monitoring alone been required. Research was therefore started into methods of building a subsection of the main computer monitoring system which could provide arrhythmia detection while conforming to the already imposed constraints of continuous real-time processing with restricted processor time and storage available, exacerbated by the requirement of multiple beds. The subsystem was to output instantaneous information about the ECG and alarms for certain potentially

126

or actually dangerous arrhythmias while providing data for time-trend analysis and displays.

A decision was reached that the easiest way to provide this subsystem would be to write a very fast screening program acting as the lowest common denominator for all beds. A much slower but much more thorough and comprehensive program could then be used to validate this program, help it when in difficulty and provide closer surveillance for critically ill patients. Work was first started on the 'screening' program. Since program speed was essential it seemed reasonable to try using a preprocessor to reduce the volume of input. All patients would have at least a bipolar chest lead with preamplifier and an electronic rate-meter. The latter device could be used to output a series of pulses indicating the relative positions of R-waves in the single-lead ECG. Thus it might be used as an analogue preprocessor to provide the computer with a series of numbers corresponding to the R-R intervals of the original ECG. It has been shown that such an interval sequence provides considerable information about heart rhythm.

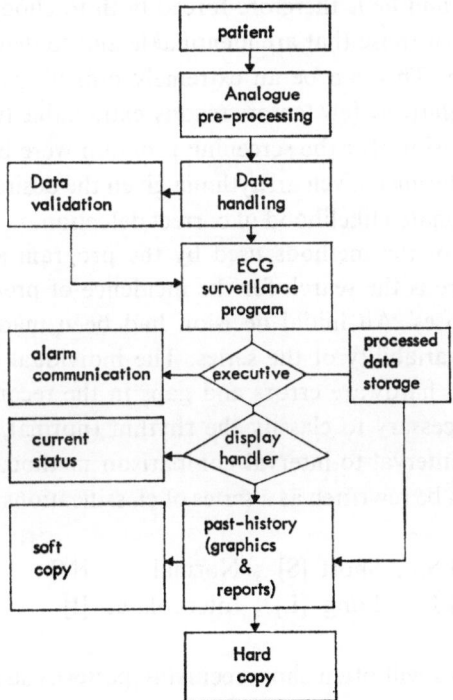

Fig. 1. Block diagram of the ECG handling subsection of the main monitoring system. Output capabilities have been included although they are, in fact, part of the main system.

A subsystem was incorporated in the main structure of the monitoring system to obtain and analyse an R-R interval series. Separate functions existed or were added for acquiring, validating, storing and analysing the data. Output was to be handled by the ordinary main-system functions giving alarms, warnings, current patient condition, time-trend graphs etc. The kernel of this subsystem is the 'screening' or analysis program. This program accepts R-R intervals singly or in groups and assumes a predecessor-successor relation between them.

The program knows nothing of multiple beds and the overhead of handling them is therefore carried by the main system which provides for swapping stored variables and buffers for different beds. The analysis is based on simple statistical principles together with simple recognition techniques which combine patterns derived from the interval series with rate and rhythm information.

The clinician should obviously play a major role in the building up of this kind of subsystem. Real-time processing rarely allows identification of all factors of interest and he is therefore forced both to choose which he needs most from the set of those that are identifiable and to determine criteria for their identification. This can be an extremely difficult problem even when dealing with the relatively few factors readily extractable from an R-R interval series. The decisions for the screening program were based on the probability of encountering a given arrhythmia given the desirability of its detection versus the estimated likelihood of correct detection.

An illustration of the methods used by the program and the reasoning behind its structure is the search for the incidence of premature beats with compensatory pauses. An initial decision had been made to estimate the current rate and variability of the series. The individual intervals were examined for certain hardware errors and gaps in the record (see appendix). It later proved necessary to classify the rhythm (normal, irregular, paired, triadic) using an interval-to-interval comparison method. With this knowledge the series can be rewritten as a series of classifications:

Extremely short [ES] ; Short [S] ; Normal   [N]
Extremely long [EL] ; Long [L] ; Interpolated [I]

This resultant series will often show recurring patterns such as the obvious:

....S ; L ; S ; L ; S....   [Bigeminy]
Taking the pattern: .... N ; S ; L ; N ....

comparison with the original series and rhythm can be used to estimate the likelihood of this pattern representing a premature beat with a partial or total compensatory pause. The majority of vPc's occurring singly (runs are treated somewhat differently) and not too late in the cycle possess full compensatory pauses. In turn, the majority of premature beats with compensatory pauses are of interest to the clinician (the majority being vPc's). Since the latter are widely recognised as being of concern to the coronary care staff as providing an early warning signal of other disorders, this arrhythmia is a typical candidate for a search.

Methods of display of quantitized and other numerical data in a clinically acceptable form are under considerable discussion at the present time. The main system provides all such display for the subsystems such as the arrhythmia detection. Immediate output takes two forms. The first is the alarms and warnings for which the upper part of the screen is reserved (fig. 2). They are

```
[14-21] ** ATTENTIE:  JANSSEN   (4.2) TACH > 110 P.MIN
          **
[14-19] ** ALARM    :  KLAASSEN (4.4)  S T I L S T A N D
---------------------------------------------------------
              CONDITIE VAN PATIENT JANSSEN (4.2)

E. C. G.      HARTSLAG            132 SLAGEN P.M
              PREMATUUR             0 LAATSTE MIN
              KORTE TACH.           0 LAATSTE 5 MIN
              DISPERSIE            12 MSECS
              PACEMAKER           GEEN PACEMAKER
              RITME               NORMAAL
              ALARMS                0 LAATSTE 5 MIN
              ATTENTIES             2 LAATSTE 5 MIN

              HAEMODYNAMICS
ARTERIEEL     RATE                ----
              SYSTOLISCH          ----
              DIASTOLISCH         ----
              ALARMS              ----
              ATTENTIES           ----

[14-23] PATIENT JANSSEN   (4.2)  TERM:4.4.0 >   1*
```

Fig. 2. The television display screen at bedside or nurse's desk showing a warning on one patient (in bed 4.2) and an alarm on another (bed 4.4). These are displayed automatically. The current patient condition with respect to the ECG is shown on request in the lower part of the screen.

displayed with classification (alarm or warning), time of occurrence and the patient's name and bed-number. Alarm display is partially controlled by priority ratings set by the clinician to ensure that the more important alarms for a particular patient are not overwritten. The remainder of the screen is used for request programs. The second form of immediate output is provided by one of these which displays current values of parameters calculated by the screening program such as heart-rate, number of premature beats etc. Further programs provide displays of time-related data, principally in the form of graphs. Time-trend graphs of parameters such as heartrate are available over periods of time between half and twenty-four hours. Hardcopy plots can also be made for inclusion in case-notes or nurses reports.

The subsystem is now under evaluation and, as the title of this lecture suggests, this is still in the very early stages. Since the normal system output is insufficiently detailed, another system function has been provided to allow a continuous dump of all relevant variables from the analysis program during normal system running. This dump is then compared on a beat-by-beat basis with a cardiologist's analysis of the corresponding electro-cardiogram tracing. This method allows considerable feed back for improvement of criteria. It is, however, slow and results are available only for the first two series of tests on 18,000 beats of 10 patients (fig. 3). Errors have been divided

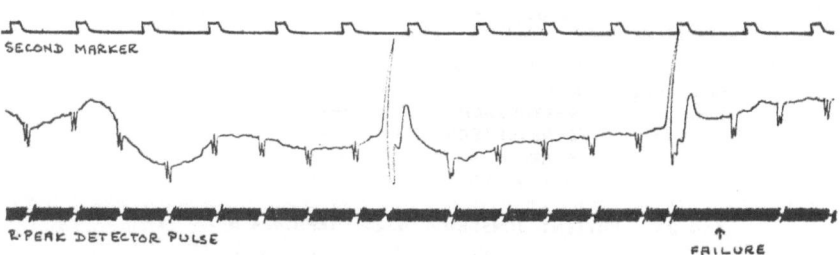

A TYPICAL PATIENT

Beat by beat analysis of computer findings compared with cardiologist's analysis of tracing.

Tracing	correct	incorrect	cause
Beats 4000			
Rhyth m Sinus	normal		
VPB's 46	42	4 (false-ve)	hardware
APB's 2	2	2 (false+ve)	software
Tachyc. 1	1	1 (false+ve)	hardware

ECG (bipolar chest lead)

SECOND MARKER

R-PEAK DETECTOR PULSE   ↑
                                        FAILURE

Portion of tracing showing VPB's, baseline drift + hardware failure.

Fig. 3. Example of evaluation of a strip chart from a patient with normal sinus rhythm and intermittent vPK's and APK's. The total record is about 1 hour.

between those caused by hardware and those caused by the program. Work is in process to improve the hardware which is, at present, unduly sensitive to muscle artifacts (fig. 4).

We are now running the system for four hours each day on one unit to accumulate more data for evaluation purposes, set up data-banks for further work and, most important of all, ascertain the feelings of the clinical staff about the methods and displays used. It seems particularly important that the program output should, in the eyes of the clinical staff, be an apt description of what they themselves see.

DETECTION RATES FOR PREMATURE BEATS
(with compensatory pauses)

1. Sinus rhythm (5) (with APB's + VPB's)			2. Atrial flutter (2)		
	incorrect	correct		incorrect	correct
positive	14	66	positive	23 ⊛	0
negative	8	11,947	negative	0	4,974

3. Atrial fibrillation (2)			4. Incomplete A-V Dissociation (1)		
	incorrect	correct		incorrect	correct
positive	1	0	positive	* 2	1
negative	0	1199	negative	0	297

Incorrect Detection	
	hardware
False+ve	12
False-ve	4
	software
False+ve	7
False-ve	4

⊛ 21 caused by intermittent variable block
* 2 atrial capture beats

Fig. 4. Results of two tests on a total of 18,000 beats on 10 patients. The error rates have been divided into those caused by hardware and those caused by software. The 21 cases of variable block have been left out of this latter subdivision since variable A-V block in atrial flutter is almost indistinguishable from a premature beat.

APPENDIX. SCREENING PROGRAM

Input is time-series of intervals analysed as such and also with simple pattern-recognition techniques.

1. Gaps in record
   sinus arrest, ecg lead fell off

5. Premature beats with partial or full compensatory pauses

2. Rate levels
   Tachycardia, bradycardia
3. Paroxysmal onset
   Tachycardias
4. Rhythm type
   Normal, irregular, paired, triplet

6. Short intervals
   very premature beats, muscle artifact
7. Premature beats (runs)
   pairs of short intervals, successive interpolated beats, short tachycardias
8. Intermittent long intervals
   Heart block, interfering rhythms, hardware errors.

REFERENCES

1. Miller, A. C., Harris, P. R., Zeelenberg, K. & Engelse, W., A multi-bed executive for an intensive care patient monitoring system, *Decus Proceedings*, Spring 1970.

2. Miller, A. C., Laird, J. D. & Hugenholtz, P. G., Computer science in the intensive care unit. Proceedings 3rd Conference *Automatic multiphase health testing*, Davos, Switzerland, September 1970.

3. Lown, B., Fakkro, A. M., Hood, W. B. & Thorn, G. W., The coronary care unit. *J. Amer. med. Ass.* 199 (1967).

METHODS FOR BEAT-TO-BEAT AND STATISTICAL CLASSIFICATION

G. VAN HERPEN, J. H. VAN BEMMEL AND C. A. SWENNE

Our interest in ECG monitoring is centered around the crucial periods of life: at it's beginning and when it is threatened in its most vital function. Monitoring provides the physician with a means on which to base his decisions. Both periods of monitoring have their own problems and difficulties, and consequently different solutions.

To monitor the foetus at birth, the heart beat of the foetus is used as a measure of foetal well-being. In this situation, one is not primarily interested in intra-cardiac conduction disturbances or congenital defects, but mainly in the regulatory aspects of the circulation and the behaviour of the control mechanism for the heart rate under different circumstances or in the event of foetal distress.

Several methods have been developed to acquire a reliable beat-to-beat foetal heart rate, with different inputs as signal source: the electrocardiogram, the phonocardiogram or ultrasonic signals (1). The main problem in foetal monitoring is that the signal-to-noise ratio is often very small, which from time to time is also a principle problem in the monitoring of ECG's from the coronary care unit.

In monitoring foetuses we were confronted with a problem comparable to that of a coronary patient: is it possible to detect gradually changing patterns in the heart rate and can we reduce the enormous amount of input data to a volume from which a human observer is able to pick up the essential aspects of the information stream? In order to reduce the large number of intervals (appr. 150 bpm), it is possible to construct interval histograms or compute mean intervals, percentile ranges, serial correlation coefficients and so on. However this entails considerable loss of information, since these heart rhythms may include slowly changing patterns as well as beat-to-beat irregularities. Both patterns may happen to have the same mean interval duration and the same frequency distribution, so that the above-mentioned data-reducing methods do not offer a means of distinguishing between the long-term irregularity and the short-term irregularity. Such distinction is retained, however, when use is made of joint interval distributions (1).

When computing scatter diagrams of consecutive intervals for a few hundred intervals (see fig. 1), one can clearly see whether the points are densely clustered around a centre (stable heart rate), clustered around a line through the origin at 45° (gradually changing heart rate) or scattered around this line (combination of irregular heart rate and long-term trends). The different patterns that may exist in such scatter diagrams can be quantified by first rotating the cluster to polar co-ordinates, i.e. by describing the position of each point by the length of its radius vector (modulus) and its angle with the abscissa (Fig. 1). The effect of this linear transformation is that short-term

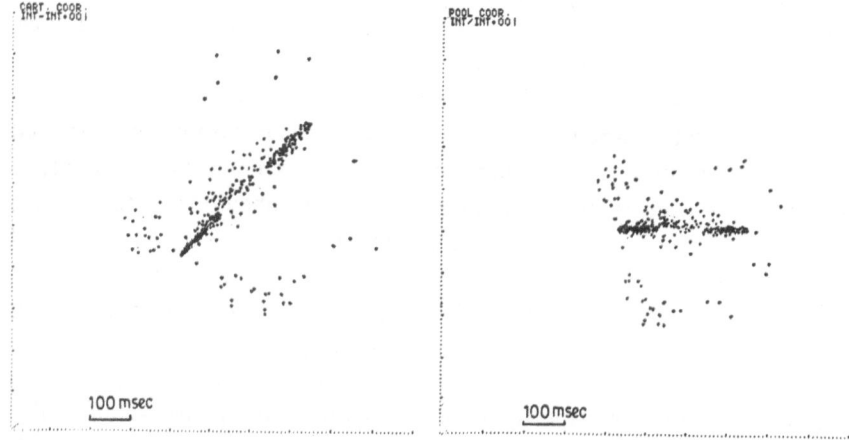

Fig. 1.
a. Scatter diagram of consecutive intervals. Most points are on a line at 45° through the origin; combinations of irregular beats are scattered around this line.
b. Transformation of figure 1a to polar co-ordinates, the ordinate being the angle and the abscissa the modulus (see text). Rapid fluctuations in interval length are most clearly seen along the angle axis and slow variations along the modulus axis.

irregularity is most clearly seen along the angle axis and long-term irregularity, along the modulus axis. Next we may further elaborate these polar scatter diagrams by constructing the projections of the cluster onto the angle axis and onto the modulus axis, so that we obtain two histograms revealing separately the frequency distributions of the short and long-term aspects respectively. In the usual interval histograms these effects are merged so that one cannot differentiate between the contributions of rapid irregularities and those of slowly changing intervals.

Such histograms of 'polar intervals' form the basis for further quantification. Percentile ranges and means can be computed so that a sequence of histograms as a function of time (minutes, hours) can reveal trends in these parameters. It appeared that especially the short-term irregularity is correlated with foetal well-being and can be used as a predictor for later foetal distress. It was also shown that this factor – which is probably the effect of a stochastic-fluctuation superimposed on the continuous vagal tone – disappears under influence of certain types of drugs given to the mother during pregnancy or birth (2).

We have also used the method of constructing scatter diagrams and their transformations to study the influence of drugs on the condition of patients in the CCU. The effect of the disappearance of arrhythmia patterns can then

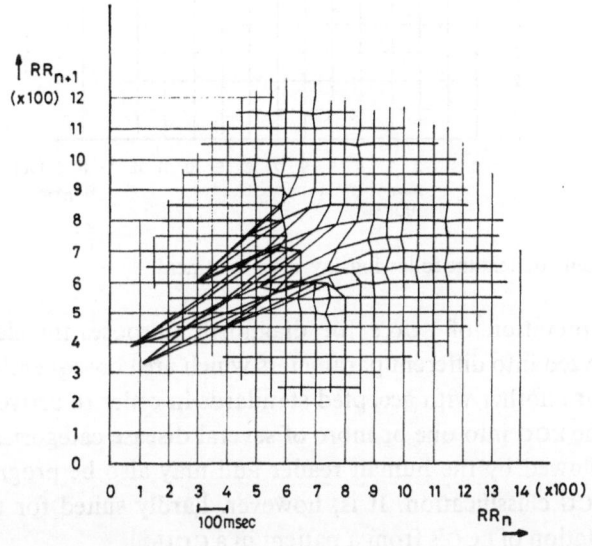

Fig. 2a. Joint interval distribution of consecutive intervals of a patient in the CCU with atrium fibrillation and unifocal extrasystoles, before treatment with pronestyl®.

be followed quantitatively day after day or hour after hour (Fig. 2). Furthermore it is an elegant means of reducing the almost infinite number of intervals received from coronary patients.

Although the statistical processing of ECG's from the CCU gives us insight into changing conditions and RR-interval patterns, it is not a method for early warning nor does it help the human operator in his fatiguing task of

observing long trains of ECG complexes on the display screen. For that
reason we, like many others (e.g. (3), (4), (5)), are searching for a method
that may assist the CCU operator in observing ECG patterns and in recognizing changes in signal shapes and intervals. The system developed starts from
the concept that every patient is his own standard of reference (6, 7).

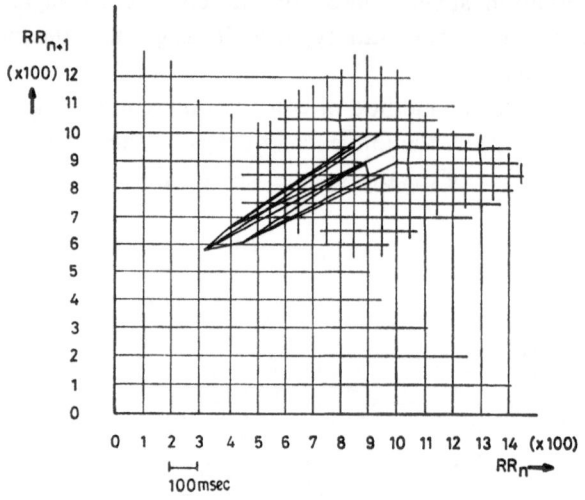

Fig. 2b. The same patient the following day, after treatment.

In the interpretation of ECG's for diagnostic purposes the electrocardiogram is analyzed into different parameters which are consequently compared
in one way or another with accepted standards in order to arrive at a classification of the ECG into one or more of several disease categories. This procedure is followed by the human reader and may also be programmed for
automatic ECG classification. It is, however, hardly suited for the analysis
and interpretation of ECG's from a patient in a CCU.

Here we usually have non-standard leads, odd wave shapes and artefacts,
and we are not primarily interested in common diagnostic statements like
anterior wall infarction or LVH. Under these circumstances no generalized or
standardized analysis is possible nor can the parameters be compared with
a set of standard parameters.

The human operator, too, has no means of diagnosing such prolonged
recordings other than comparison of each new heart beat with previous
beats from the same patient. Therefore he needs some time, after the connection of the patient to the electrodes, to 'learn' what types of patterns belong

to this patient. With the help of these patterns, stored on a CRT, on paper or in his mind, he is then able to compare different ECG complexes.

We have set up a processing system which 'simulates' the recognition sequence followed by the human operator. Our system therefore has many interactive features: the human operator 'teaches' the computer the different patterns, whereas the computer 'asks' the operator for intervention when it cannot find the solution to a problem of ECG recognition.

Although at present the system runs off-line from magnetic tape and the entire processing is done digitally in the computer, our plan is for a large portion of the analysis to be done by pre-processing equipment in an on-line environment. The sequence of the processing and decision steps can be seen in figure 3.

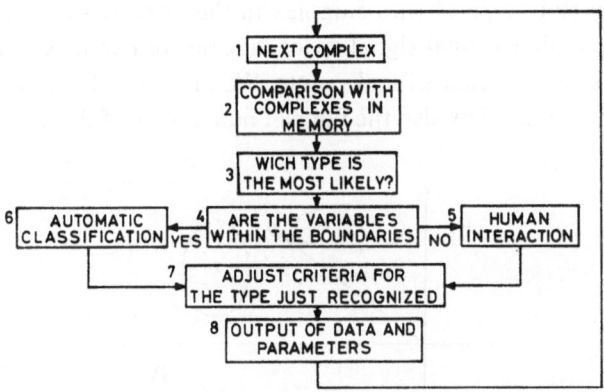

Fig. 3. Decision scheme of interactive program for QRS classification. In the different stages, the following operations are performed:

1. Filtering, QRS detection, point of reference, parameters
2. Measurement of distances to clusters
3. Compute minimal distance
4. Compare with threshold
5. Accept or reject pattern. If accepted, then classify it in one of the categories or define a new cluster.
6. Accept pattern and give warning if certain criteria are not met.
7. Adjust means and variances. Go in adaptive mode if desired.
8. Give output of trends and statistics.

The first step after the input stage of the ECG into the computer is the detection of ventricular complexes. This is done with the help of a digital band pass-filter between 6 and 40 Hz. After QRS finding and the computation of a reference point in the filtered QRS complex, the data are reduced to only 8 samples at 13.3 msec intervals. Already at this stage the human operator has to make decisions, it is up to him to determine what parts of the QRS complex to the left and to the right of the point of reference are most relevant for type definition of that complex. Once the operator has done so, the complex is stored into the memory in the form of the 8 amplitudes mentioned. These parameters thus form the base for the recognition of subsequent complexes of the same type. For every new type, a new base is formed by human intervention. In this way, every new complex is taught to the computer.

If we only use the shape of the complex as a measure for recognition, only the first beat per type is needed for later comparison, e.g. by cross-correlation methods. We felt however that it was important to use not only the shape, i.e. the amplitudes, but also the variances as measures for recognition. If we represent a certain type of QRS complex in the ECG by the end point of a vector in the 8-dimensional signal space, a series of complexes of the same type gives rise to a cluster of end points. We are then able to compute not only the gravity point but also the fiducial boundaries of the cluster (Fig. 4).

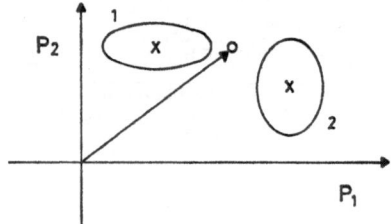

Fig. 4. Two-dimensional representation of clusters for two wave shapes. When an unknown vector falls within the boundaries of one of the clusters, it is recognized automatically; if not, human intervention is requested.

A new QRS-complex is then required to fall within the boundaries of one of the clusters if it is to be accepted automatically as a member of the family. If it does not do so, the operator is asked by the computer for human intervention. The operator is then still free to allocate the complex to an existing cluster or to start a new type of cluster. If he decides on the first course, he will thereby widen the boundaries of the cluster of his choice and thus increase the variances.

The program has been set-up such that after a given learning period and once automatic recognition starts, the criteria – means, variances and boundaries – are continuously and automatically adapted to slow changes in the QRS patterns.

The more stable and noise-free a QRS shape is, the narrower the boundaries for classification are, so that a strange wave shape is almost certainly identified. The adaptive phase starts after 20 complexes have been seen by the computer, either by teaching or automatically.

The effect of learning is shown in figure 5 where one can see the decreasing

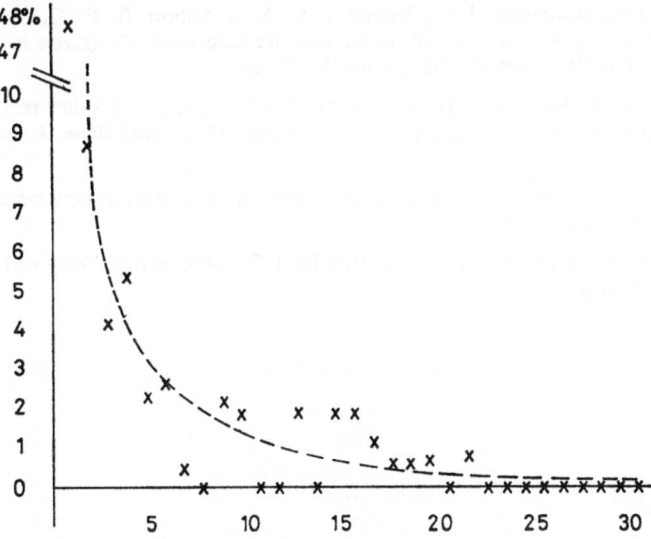

Fig. 5. Decreasing percentage of human interactions as a function of learning. The percentage of taught complexes is given along the vertical axis per group of 20 complexes and the time or the number of groups, along the horizontal axis.

percentage of human intervention as time proceeds. The total number of human interferences are represented per group of 20 beats for 10 different patients with up to 5 different complexes.

The main advantage of the method is the fact that it is not fully independent, but open for human interaction. The principal advantage of such systems is that they do not have to take over human tasks completely but they can liberate the human operator from the tiring work of having to observe the ECG on a monitor screen, giving him time to care for the source of the information, the patient.

REFERENCES

1. Van Bemmel, J. H., *Detection and processing of foetal ECG's*. Nijmegen 1969.

2. De Haan, J., et al., Quantitative analysis of fetal heart rate patterns. *Europ. J. Obst. Gynec.* 3, 4, 96, 137 (1971).

3. Cox, J. R., Nolle, F. M., Fozzard, H. A. & Oliver, G. C., Aztec, a preprocessing program for real-time ECG rhythm analysis. *IEEE Trans. Biom. Engng.* 15, 128 (1968).

4. Osborn, J. J., Beaumont, J. O., Raison, J. C. A. & Abbott, R. P., Computation for quantitative on-line measurements in an intensive care ward. *Computers in Biomedical Research*. Vol. III. p. 207-237. New York (N.Y.) 1969.

5. Haywood, L. J., Murthy, V. K., Harvey, G. A. & Saltzberg, S., On-line real time computer algorithm for monitoring the ECG waveform. *Comp. and Biom. Research*. 3, 15 (1970).

6. Swenne, C. A., *A study relating to the classification of ventricle complexes in the ECG* (in Dutch). Eindhoven 1971.

7. Swenne, C. A., et al., Pattern recognition for ECG monitoring. *Comp and Biom. Research* (in press).

DISCUSSION

Van Bemmel: I wonder if Miss Hoare could tell us a bit more about what she considers the main problem in the automated quantitative analysis of cardiac rhythm.

Hoare: I find that almost unanswerable. The problems are as many as the doctors and the units involved. There are the problems of finance, computer time and deciding what you want as output. Most important, we do not yet know how we should handle arrhythmia analysis or arrhythmia monitoring. We think it best to look for ventricular premature beats, the nature of the rhythm, etc. There are however all sorts of possibilities. Possibly the right method will resemble what Prof. Sayers was talking about earlier. In fact, I feel certain that in the future this is the way we must proceed – to find parameters which tell us more about how the patient is actually doing, not about the specific arrhythmia he is suffering from.

Van Bemmel: I would like Mr. Neilson to comment on what parameters we should look for in our cardiac rhythm recordings and what parameters will be most important in the future.

Neilson: At the moment most of us are working on some aspects of research into the arrhythmias but this is not an end in itself. As I see it, this is going to lead to the assessment of a technique of management, different drugs etc. Once the results of clinical research (cf. my previous paper) are known, and once we know which arrhythmias are urgent and important, the problem will be to detect them. Therefore, I think that there will always be a place for some kind of machinery to help the clinical staff. There are still some difficult technical problems. Excluding economic and financial aspects, the biggest problem is the signal-to-noise ratio. The ECG's that we get in the monitoring situation are not the classical ECG's as the clinicians usually see. You would be horrified if you saw a 24 hr recording. But those are the kind of signals that the machinery has to deal with.

Van Herpen: I don't think that you should ask the physicists, engineers or technical people what to do with the signals and what to do about arrhythmia analysis. I would like to hear something from the audience. They should state what they are interested in; then the technical people should provide them with the means and the tools to find out.

Sayers: I should like to make a brief remark about the last comment with which I totally and flatly disagree. We are in a situation where we do not have sufficient information to provide a basis to define what we need to do. I think at the moment we need to orientate ourselves with respect to the sort of data that we will be able to get from the patient. I think that there is a task for the technologists and the physicists here to provide us with a data base.

On the other hand we have to use our limited insight into the pathophysiology to decide what it is broadly speaking that we should be looking for; then we must acquire the necessary information and from that take the next clinical steps.

Van Herpen: My remark was meant of course to trigger discussion. Everything should be interactive. We are at the stage now where we have offered something, even though it is very little. Now, the clinician should comment on those aspects presented here which he considers useful.

Snellen: In general terms you could say that we are interested in prediction. We should like to know if you could show us what precedes the events which we already know to be potentially or actually dangerous. For example: it is surprising to cardiologists that a faster rhythm should produce more extrasystoles, as Mr. Neilson showed in one of his slides.

Neilson: I hope I made it clear that this particular slide was only one patient which I presented just to show you that matters are not always as simple as they are supposed to be. Perhaps there is something strange about this patient's vagal connections to his heart. It certainly is an exception.

Comment from the audience (Meurs): We examined 100 patients with an acute infarction for 72 hours. There were some with brachycardia, which we defined as a sinus rhythm below 50. These patients had no more, or even less, ventricular extrasystoles than the other patients. We therefore think that the hypothesis that bradycardia predisposes to ventricular extrasystoles is unproven.

Neilson: If I may take up the previous point once again, I must say that I feel a bit confused. Since we are all disagreeing flatly about things, may I in turn disagree flatly with prof. Sayers' remark that we do not know what we want to do. I must be in the wrong world if that is true. There are certain things that need to be done right now. That is automation of what is now done by oscilloscopes and nurses on shifts around the clock. By ordinary visual observation you cannot say with certainty that out of the 200,000 complexes that a patient has in two days none is a 'R or T'. So we are missing a great deal that actually happens. It would be very nice if we could reach the stage where we can predict half a day in advance that a patient is going into ventricular fibrillation, but we have a big job ahead just handling the problems already with us.

CHAPTER 5

LEFT VENTRICULAR FUNCTION

THE SIGNIFICANCE OF MEASUREMENT OF
CONTRACTILITY OF THE HEART

D. L. BRUTSAERT

The circulation of blood through the vascular system is maintained by the rhythmic contraction of the heart. This pumping action depends on the ability of its muscular fibres to develop force and to shorten. An important development in our understanding of cardiac physiology has been the consideration of the heart as a muscle in order to gain greater insight into the operation of the heart as a pump.

The basic principles of the mechanics of skeletal muscle contraction have been studied thoroughly over the past forty years. In contrast, these principles have only been applied to cardiac muscle in the past decade and their application has been useful in the evaluation of the contractile function of the intact normal and diseased heart in man.

I. BASIC PROPERTIES: FORCE-VELOCITY-LENGTH-TIME RELATIONSHIPS

Figure 1 illustrates a classical experiment of muscle physiology, performed on an isolated papillary muscle of the right ventricle of the cat. In the upper section, shortening, velocity of shortening, and developed force are shown for 6 twitch contractions selected from a series of isotonic contractions. From left to right these are a nonafterloaded contraction at a preload of 0.4 g, four contractions at increasing afterloads and a complete isometric contraction. The peak velocities of shortening for these contractions are plotted in the lower section, as a function of total load. The values obtained at intermediate afterloads, which are not represented in the upper section, are also included. This inverse relationship between velocity of shortening and load represents the most fundamental and generally accepted feature of active muscle.

From the experiment shown in figure 1, it is clear that this force-velocity relationship can also be applied to some extent to *twitch* contractions of heart muscle. Moreover, in figure 2 it will be demonstrated that this curve for heart muscle, like that for skeletal muscle, corresponds to a hyperbola, at least for the lightest loads, and can also be described by the Hill equation.

However, mainly due to the fact that heart muscle cannot be tetanized under normal conditions (1), two additional variables have to be considered

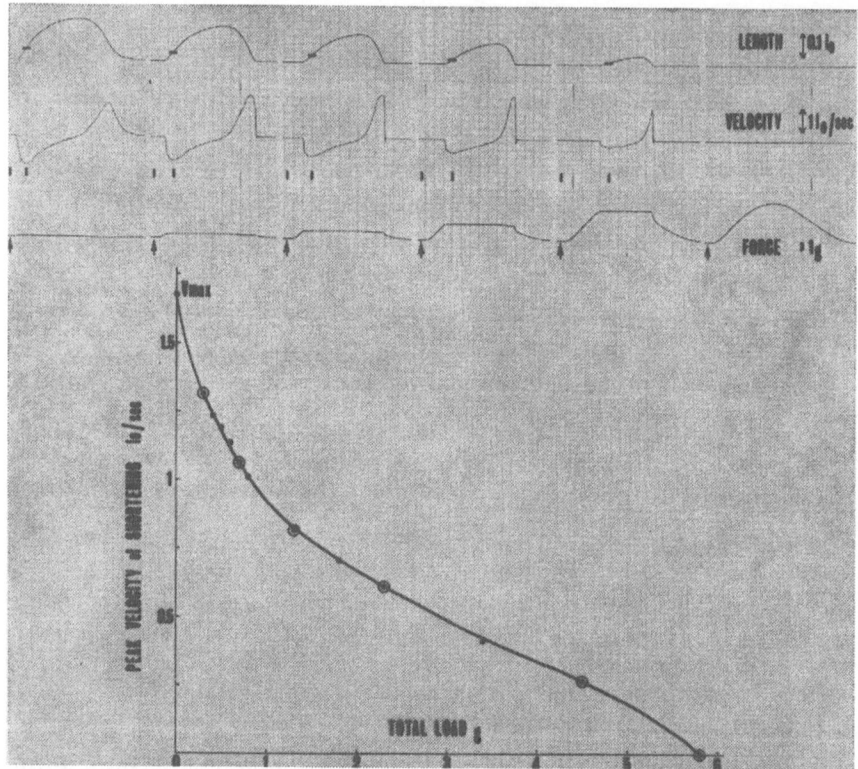

Fig. 1. Upper section: shortening, velocity of shortening and developed force of a series of contractions of a cat papillary muscle. The length, at which peak velocity occurs, is indicated by the horizontal dash on the shortening tracing, while the time after the stimulation is indicated by a vertical dash.
Lower section: peak velocity of shortening as a function of total load (force-peak velocity curve). Temp. 29° C; 12/min.; cross-sectional area 0.99 mm².

in the analysis of *twitch* contractions of heart muscle. The first variable deals with the *muscle length* at which peak velocity of shortening is measured during shortening. Indeed, in the experiment of figure 1, there is a difference in length of 5-6% between contractions 1 and 5. The second variable deals with the *time* lapse between the stimulus and the peak velocity. It becomes evident from figure 1 that each point of a force-velocity curve for twitch

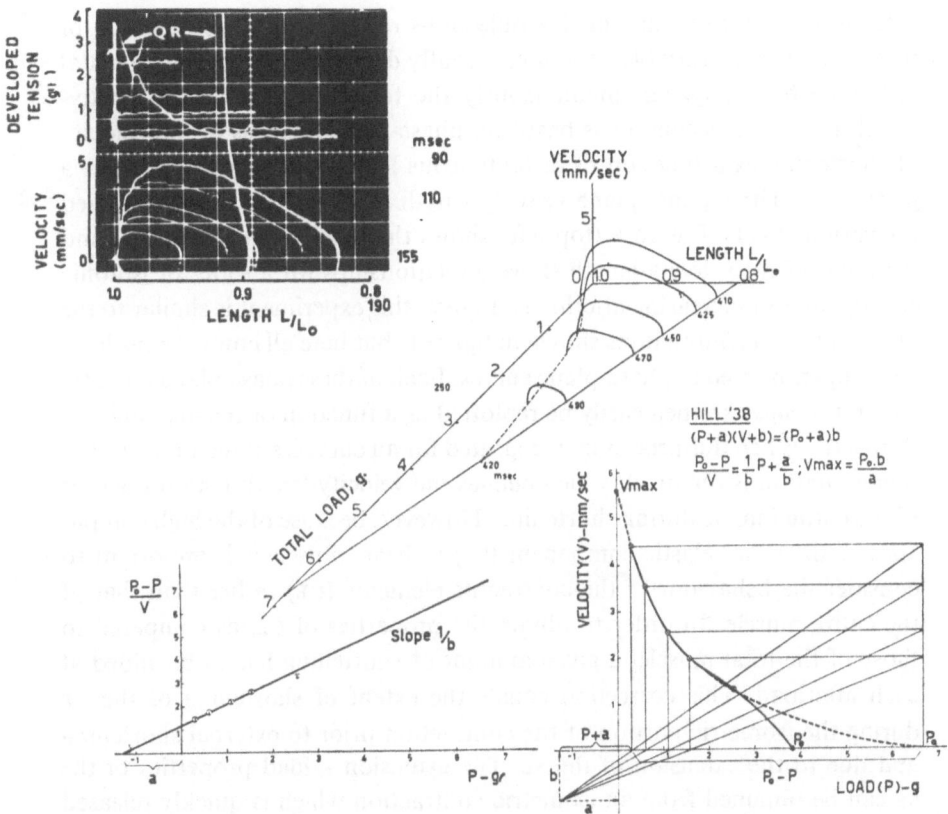

Fig. 2. Force-velocity-length relationships of a cat papillary muscle.

Top left: tension-length and phase-plane velocity-length tracings of total muscle during isotonic contractions at increasing afterloads. See text.

Top right: from the phase-plane tracings a three-dimensional graph is constructed with correction for the SE. See text. Times from stimulation to peak velocity are indicated on the left, and times to peak shortening and to peak tension on the right. The extrapolation of the linear load-shortening relationship for the CE permits an estimation of the maximum isometric force (P_0) of the CE at that precise length if there were no extension of the SE. This procedure can only be done for small preloads (e.g. $\leqslant 0.5$ g/mm²), where the extrapolation to the theoretical P_0 is still measured in the ascending portion of the length-tension relationship for the CE.

Bottom right: the force peak velocity relationship for the CE is hyperbolic at the lightest loads, when corrected to this force P_0. The Hill constants a and b can be determined either graphically (right) or after linearization of the Hill equation (left).

Preload 0.3 g; cross-sectional area 0.98 mm²; L_0 4.82 mm; temp. 29° C; frequency 12/min. Reproduced by permission form *Circulat. Res.*

contractions in heart muscle is measured at different time intervals after the onset of activation.

In order to answer the possible objections raised by the consideration of these 2 additional variables, we have recently developed a new experimental technique for analyzing simultaneously the four variables, force-velocity-length-time. This technique is based on phase-plane analysis of the velocity of shortening as a function of instantaneous length during shortening at a given load. These phase-plane velocity-length relations can then be studied for various loads. Figure 2 (top left) shows the tension-length (upper) and the phase-plane velocity-length (lower) relationships for a series of isotonic contractions at increasing afterloads. In fact, this experiment is similar to the series of twitch contractions shown in figure 1, but here all contractions have been superimposed as phase-plane curves. Each of these phase-plane velocity-length tracings can then easily be replotted as a function of the load along a third axis. When this procedure is repeated for all curves, a three-dimensional representation is obtained, which defines the velocity-length-load properties of the entire muscle during shortening. However, because of the high compliance of the series elastic component (SE) in heart muscle it is important to consider the behaviour of the contractile elements (CE) rather than that of the entire muscle. In order to obtain the properties of CE, as compared to those of the total muscle, a given amount of shortening has to be added at each afterload. This correction equals the extent of shortening of the CE during the isometric portion of the contraction prior to external shortening and due to the extension of the SE. The extension – load properties of the SE can be obtained from an isometric contraction which is quickly released at various loads. In figure 2 (top left) the tension-length (left arrow) and velocity-length (right arrow) relationships for such quick release (QR) from peak tension to zero afterload is superimposed on all tracings. In the middle of figure 2, a three-dimensional graph of the velocity-length relationship is constructed after correction for the extension of the SE, thus describing the force-velocity relationship of the muscle as a function of the change in length of the CE during isotonic muscle shortening.

In the contractions of figure 1, peak velocity of shortening was attained at progressively longer muscle lengths as the load was increased. Hence, it could be argued that discrepancies relative to the length-tension relationship of the muscle might occur, if velocity were greatly dependent on length. However during the isometric portion of these contractions, the CE had shortened at the expense of the SE so that the CE length did not correspond to the muscle length. In the experiment shown in Fig. 2 it is striking that the peak velocity of each phase-plane velocity-length tracing on the three-dimensional diagram corrected for SE occurs at the same CE length within a range of 1 to 1.5% L_0. Hence, although it is obvious from the phase-plane analysis that the velocity of shortening at any given load is determined by the instantaneous length, it is equally clear that the 'peak' velocity values, and therefore the entire force-peak velocity curve of figure 1, are measured at nearly the same CE length.

It has been claimed that the active state in heart muscle has a rather slow onset and reaches a maximum only late during the contraction (2, 3, 4, 5). From this view, it has been deduced that peak velocity of shortening for light loads would be measured at a time when the active state is not yet at a maximum. Thus, the portion of the force-velocity curve at the light loads would be underestimated. However, in contrast to previous literature, we feel that we have gathered enough recent evidence to postulate an early onset of the active state, followed by a plateau during a great portion of the contraction. These findings are of utmost importance since the application of this force-velocity relationship to heart muscle can only be valid if the activating substance or the active state is maintained at a constant level.

Arguments for an early onset and subsequent plateau of active state over a great portion of the shortening phase of the contraction in heart muscle will be given in the next experiments. In figure 3 the phase-plane velocity-length relationships for 9 isotonic contractions have been superimposed. Shortening was initiated for 9 different initial lengths with the same total load. Hence, all 9 contractions occur in the same vertical transsection of the three-dimensional diagram of figure 2. In each contraction, velocity of shortening rises to a common velocity-length relationship. Thus, velocity of shortening for a given total load is a unique function of instantaneous length during shortening, regardless of the initial length from which the muscle starts to shorten and also independent of the time between the onset of shortening and close-to-peak shortening. For example, at the length indicated by the arrow the first 7 contractions shorten at the same speed despite a difference in time up to 65 msec. From these findings it is clear that the three-dimensional surface described by the force-velocity-length relationships is largely independent of time, except somewhat prior to peak shortening. Along the terminal portion of shortening the velocity-length relationships in figure 3 clearly dissociate, due to limitations in time. However, it could also be theorized that such precise interrelations of force, velocity and length during the phase of contraction between onset of shortening and peak shortening might be a coincidence due to a slowly increasing intensity of active state and a decre-

asing muscle length (6). In recent experiments in our laboratory a new technique has been designed, in which sudden alterations of load were imposed
during the course of isotonic shortening between the onset of shortening and
peak shortening. The results obtained with this 'load clamping' technique

Constant total load – 0.35 g
Muscle length (at 0.35 g preload) - L_O – 6.2 mm
Temperature – 29 °C
Frequency – 12/min

Time after stimulus (msec)

1	175
2	170
3	160
4	150
5	140
6	125
7	110

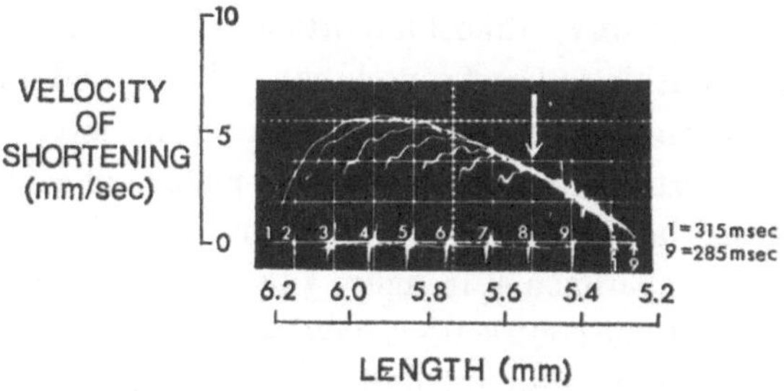

Fig. 3. Phase-plane velocity-length tracings of 9 isotonic contractions at the same total
load. The phase of relaxation is not displayed. See text. Reproduced by permission from
Circulat. Res.

provide additional irrefutable arguments to postulate the time independence
of the force-velocity-length relationships. The original study (7) should be
consulted for more details. A representative example of such experiments is
illustrated in figure 4. In section A, the phase-plane recording of velocity of
shortening as a function of length for 5 isotonic contractions has been corrected for series elastic extension and replotted as a function of total load. In
this manner, a three-dimensional relationship between force-velocity and
length has been constructed for the contractile element. When the load is abruptly altered, i.e. between B-C-D-E, the velocity rapidly adjusts according
to the load and length, independent of time. For example at length X in section B, the same velocity of shortening is reached in the control and clamped contractions at each load despite substantial differences in time after

stimulation (section C). The deviation in velocities in the terminal portion of the shortening (E to F) is due to limitations in time when peak shortening is approached and the active state may start to decline. Were force and velocity to be plotted as a function of time, a unique surface such as noted above

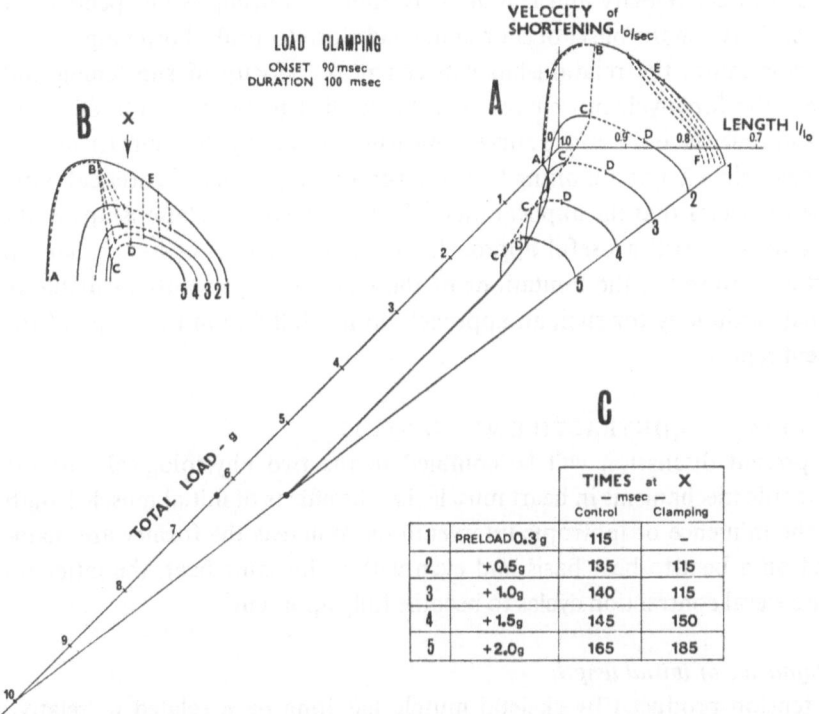

Fig. 4. The force-velocity-length relationships for the contractile elements of a cat papillary muscle. In section A, the phase-plane relationships of velocity as a function of length for 5 contractions have been plotted as a function of total load. The starting point for each contraction on the basis of length versus load has been corrected for the extension of the series elastic component (SE). The load-extension curve of the SE was determined by a quick release from peak isometric force (18, 19). Section B shows the same phase-plane tracings displaced to correct for the SE. The arrow beneath the X points to a selected common length at which the times have been measured as shown in section C for both the control and clamped contractions. Muscle cross-sectional area 0.55 mm². Lo, length with 0.3 preload is 7.33 mm. The time to peak isometric force of an isometric contraction at the preload of 0.3 g was 360 msec.

could not be obtained. Similar observations were made for various loads, regardless of whether the muscle was loaded or unloaded, and also independent of the time at which the load alteration had been imposed between the onset of shortening and close-to-peak shortening. These results imply that the active state in heart muscle sets in early in the course of the contraction and is maintained at a constant level throughout the major portion of shortening.

In summary, the mechanical performance of twitch contractions of heart muscle can be defined entirely by the surface described by the relationship between force, velocity and length. This interrelationship is independent of the time between the onset of shortening and close-to-peak shortening.

Furthermore, the relationship between peak velocity of shortening and force – the force-velocity curve – can be applied to twitch contractions in heart muscle since the entire curve is measured at nearly the same CE length, and since time is not a limiting factor. Accordingly, from a theoretical point of view it seems that the application of the force-velocity relationships to the intact heart is still a useful approach for the evaluation of its mechanical function. However, the limitations of the techniques presently available in clinical cardiology for such an approach do not fall within the scope of the present report.

II. VARIABLE CONTRACTILE MECHANISMS

The present discussion will be confined to the two physiological variable contractile mechanisms in heart muscle, i.e. the effects of initial muscle length and the influence of inotropic interventions. Whereas the former are manifested on a beat-to-beat basis and even within the same beat, the latter require several contraction cycles to become fully apparent.

A. Influence of initial length

The tension produced by skeletal muscle has long been related to relative muscle length (8). More recently, tension developed and maximum velocity of shortening have been ascribed to length-dependent properties of the sarcomere (12). From the work of these authors on skeletal muscle fibers, it has become clear that both active tetanic force developed and the maximum velocity of shortening under unloaded conditions remain constant for sarcomere lengths between 2.25 and 1.95 μ. Over this range of lengths the overlap between actin and myosin filaments is optimal, i.e. a maximum number of crossbridges can be activated. At shorter sarcomere lengths both force and velocity decrease; the reasons for this phenomenon are not really understood, but include double overlap of thin filaments, restoring forces (9), greater separation of thick and thin filaments (10) and a poorly defined process of inactivation (11, 12). At longer lengths, active tetanic force development decreases linearly with increasing length. This diminishing force is to be expected on the basis of the decreasing degree of overlap and hence the lower number of active sites acting in parallel. In contrast, maximum velocity of shortening under unloaded conditions remains constant independent of the sarcomere length after 2.25 μ, and hence clearly dissociates from the length-tension relationship. These findings provide an ultrastructural basis for the sliding filament theory of Huxley (13), in which force represents the number of contractile sites activated while V_{max} reflects the maximum rate of turn-over for one contractile site independent of the number activated and of time.

A similar relationship between length and mechanical performance is also manifested in twitch contractions of heart muscle and has long been known as the Frank Starling Law of the Heart. In view of the current opinions on skeletal muscle summarized above, this Law of the Heart was re-analyzed in our laboratory in an attempt to explain the many discrepancies found in recent literature on heart muscle.

In recent studies (14) the force-velocity-length relationships were analyzed under no-load conditions. These unloading experiments were performed using a new method by which the preload is removed during the course of shortening and the maximal velocity of shortening (V_{max}) of the contractile elements is measured directly (Fig. 5). This value is maintained at a constant

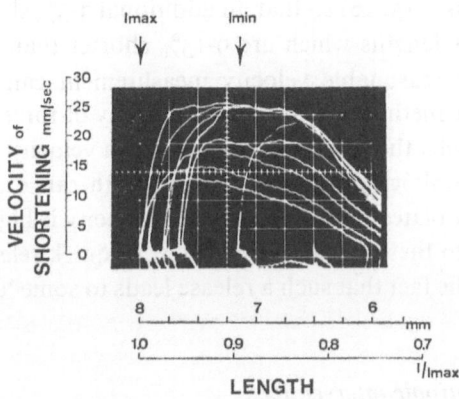

Fig. 5. Unloading of a cat papillary muscle during shortening. Velocity of shortening is displayed as a function of length during shortening of five non-afterloaded isotonic contractions which started shortening from five different initial muscle lengths. The preloads were from left to right, 0.7 g (L_{max}), 0.5 g, 0.3 g, 0.2 g and 0.1 g (L_{min}); L_{min} indicates the length at the lowest possible preload in this muscle. The preload was removed during shortening according to the resting length-tension relationships for the same muscle. Superimposed are the velocity-length relationships for the five control contractions in which the preload was maintained constant throughout shortening (five lower curves). 29° C; 12/min. Cross-sectional area 0.56 mm².

level from the length at which the active force is a maximum (L_{max}) until
L_{max}-minus-12.5%. This range encompasses the sarcomere lengths between
2.2 and 1.9 μ.

Accordingly, one could conclude that over the physiological range of
initial muscle and sarcomere lengths, where myofilament overlap is optimal,
the maximum velocity of shortening under unloading conditions remains relatively independent of length. These results are in agreement with the results
of Gordon et al. (9) for skeletal muscle fibers. However, since sarcomeres of
heart muscle are remarkably resistant to acute as well as chronic overstretch
and never exceed lengths of approximately 2.2 μ, sarcomere lengths longer
than l_{Max} (approximately 2.2 μ) cannot be explored in heart muscle. Also
in good agreement with the findings obtained in skeletal muscle (9) is the
decrease in the maximum velocity of shortening under unloading conditions
in the short length range below L_{max} – minus – 12.5%, i.e. less than approximately 1.9 μ. This observation largely explains the discrepancies with recent
findings in literature obtained with quick release techniques (5). If an isome-
trically contracting muscle is released to the preload after at least 25-50% of
the time to peak tension, the CE will have already shortened 5-10% of their
initial length before the release due to the SE extension. Moreover, a finite
interval of time is needed for the release itself and for velocity transients
following the release (15, 16) so that an additional 3-5% shortening of the CE
occurs. This yields lengths which are 9-15% shorter than the initial muscle
length before any reasonable velocity measurement can be made. Hence
when quick release methods are used for the study of force-velocity relationships in heart muscle, the values of the maximum velocity of shortening will
be obtained in the short non-physiological length range on the right-hand
side of the velocity plateau, where maximum velocity is highly length-dependent. In addition to these obvious limitations of quick release, another difficulty arises from the fact that such a release leads to some 'uncoupling' of the
active state.

B. Influence of inotropic interventions

Mammalian heart is able to modify its performance over a very large scale,
independent of its filling conditions and hence of the initial length of its individual fibers. A great variety of these influences have long been described as
so-called 'positive inotropic' interventions or 'potentiating' mechanisms of
the heart (17), e.g. the influence of the frequency of the heartbeat (frequency
potentiation, Bowditch staircase or Treppe Phenomenon), the effects of a
single (postextrasystolic potentiation) or of a series of sustained extrabeats

(paired stimulation potentiation), the influence of temperature, of calcium ions and of pharmacological agents (catecholamines, digitalis derivatives, etc.). On the other hand depression of heart muscle function, such as occurs in heart failure, is known as a so-called 'negative inotropic' phenomenon. All these interventions represent mechanisms which interfere either directly or indirectly with the intrinsic activation system of the contractile machinery.

The present study deals with a more thorough descriptive analysis of the mechanical aspects of these inotropic interventions based on newer techniques recently developed in our laboratory. An attempt will be made to provide an unifying concept of the force-velocity-length-time relationships in heart muscle.

The effects of an augmented calcium concentration as seen in figure 6 provide a representative example of a positive inotropic intervention. The entire force-velocity-length surface of the CE is shifted upwards in comparison to the control conditions, so that the velocity of shortening is augmented at any CE length and load. When a steady state is reached the surface is again unique for this particular state of contractility, regardless of the initial muscle length (18, 19) and also regardless of the time for the major portion of shortening as shown in load clamping experiments.

Thus, the force-velocity-length relationships of the CE offer a most valuable dynamic approach to the study of the effects of various inotropic interventions. Changes in the filling conditions of the heart or in the initial time range for the active state do not alter conclusions. As with calcium, observations and conclusions can be made for all known positive inotropic interventions in heart muscle. Moreover with increasing afterloads, the peak velocity values occur at nearly the same CE length as under control conditions so that the force-peak velocity curves are directly comparable for all inotropic interventions.

As pointed out in previous studies on the force-velocity relationships in heart muscle (20, 17), the effects of inotropic agents on peak tension are not necessarily as marked as the effects on velocity values at smaller loads. This explains why for any given initial muscle length either a symmetrical (post-extrasystolic and paired stimulation potentiation, calcium, digitalis) or an asymmetrical (temperature, frequency potentiation, isoproterenol) shift of the force-velocity curve may ensue. This observation implies that the maximum velocity of shortening, the extrapolation of these curves to zero load, would always be increased during any positive inotropic intervention. For this precise reason V_{max} has been proposed as a useful index in cardiology to distinguish between alterations in myocardial performance due to inotropic interventions and those due to changes in filling conditions (20). Indeed, from peak velocity measurements (20, 17) phase plane analysis (18) or unloading experiments (see part 1) under the latter conditions, it appears that V_{max} is

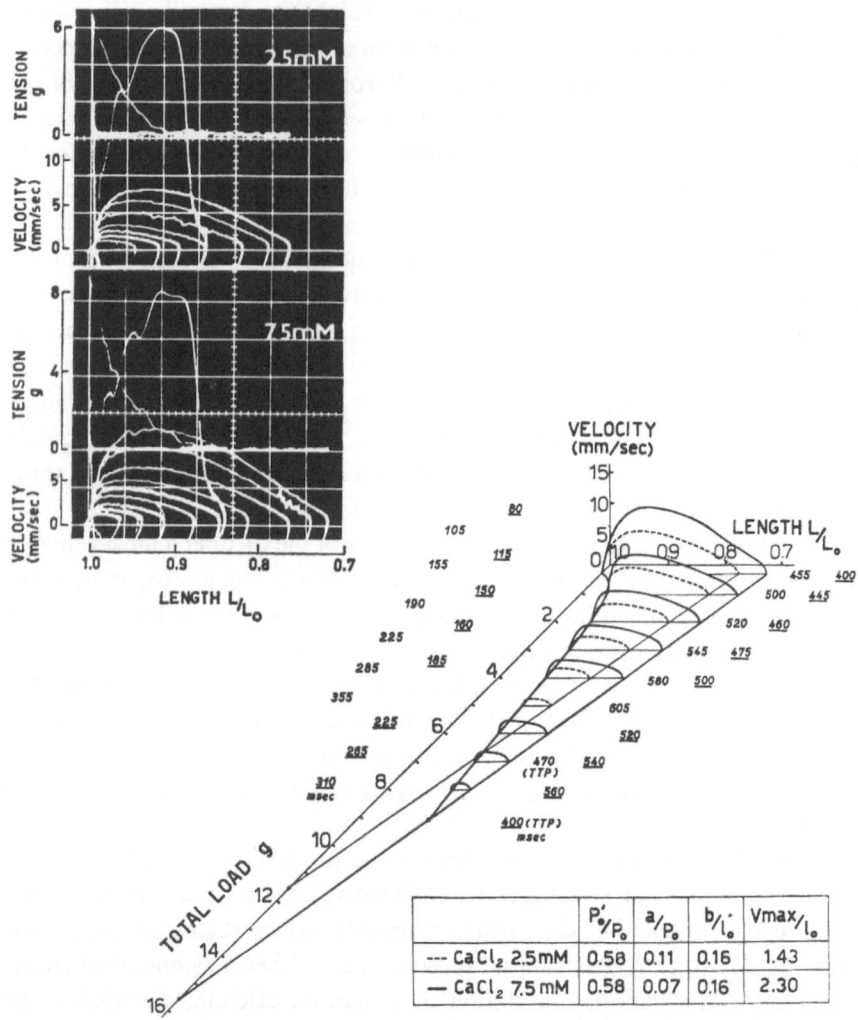

	P'_o/P_o	a/P_o	b/l_o	$Vmax/l_o$
--- CaCl₂ 2.5mM	0.58	0.11	0.16	1.43
— CaCl₂ 7.5 mM	0.58	0.07	0.16	2.30

Fig. 6. Effects of two calcium concentrations (2.5 and 5.0 mM/l) on the three-dimensional force-velocity-length relationships for the contratile elements. The tracings in the upper left were obtained as in figure 3. The dynamic constants as derived from the Hill equation are shown in the insert. Times from stimulation to peak velocities are indicated on the left, and times to peak shortening and to peak isometric tension (TTP) are indicated on the right. Muscle length (L₀) 6.0 mm at preload of 0.3 g; cross-sectional area 0.67 mm².Reproduced by permission from *Circulat. Res.*

barely modified by changes in initial muscle length within the range of physiological lengths, whereas under the former conditions this parameter always differs markedly.

On the other hand Katz (21) has challenged the observation that V_{max} of the CE is truly elevated under the former conditions. This author has emphasized the fact that the pure actomyosin system is not altered by calcium but its inhibition by troponin is removed by this ion. Thus, if calcium does not affect the actin and myosin interaction directly but only binds to troponin (22), it is hard to see how it can alter the intrinsic rate of the crossbridge interaction. Alternatively, how can calcium levels alter V_{max}? One would expect calcium availability to change tension development while V_{max} remains unaltered.

Thus is V_{max} actually altered when calcium levels are changed, or is the mechanical measurement itself, as derived from extrapolated force-velocity curves, unreliable or subject to error due to an unrecognized internal load?

With these considerations in mind, we have directly measured maximum velocity of shortening during positive inotropic interventions using the 'unloading' technique. Again, calcium was taken as a representative positive inotropic intervention; the results are illustrated in figure 7. In the upper and middle sections, the length-tension relationships are shown for calcium levels of 2.5 and 5.0 mM. The longest initial length taken was just beyond the point of maximum developed tension (L_{max}). With high calcium, peak developed tension is enhanced at each length as compared to low calcium. The resting tension curve is unaltered and the resting tension at l_{max} is only 10-15% of the total developed tension. In the lower section, the phase-plane velocity-length relationships of four isotonic contractions are shown. In all four contractions, shortening starts from L_{max}. The two lower tracings represent the isotonic control contractions at 2.5 and 5.0 mM calcium where the preload was maintained throughout shortening. As demonstrated previously in figure 6, the velocity of shortening is increased at all lengths for high calcium. In the two upper tracings, the contractions start shortening with the same preload, but the preload has been removed progressively during the course of shortening. This unloading has been described in figure 5 and is performed according to the resting length-tension relation as shown in the upper two sections. For high calcium, the maximum velocity of shortening under unloading conditions is higher at all lengths. This relative increase in maximum velocity for high calcium as compared to the velocity for low calcium, both under unloaded conditions, is somewhat greater than the relative increase in the preloaded isotonic control contraction. This finding supports the view that the force-velocity relationships at all lengths are altered and cannot be convergent toward zero load. This would mean that the increased maximum velocity of shortening for high calcium is indeed truly elevated. In more recent experiments it has been demonstrated that this calcium dependence cannot be explained by an internal load (23). Moreover, regardless of the contractile state, the unloaded velocity of shortening

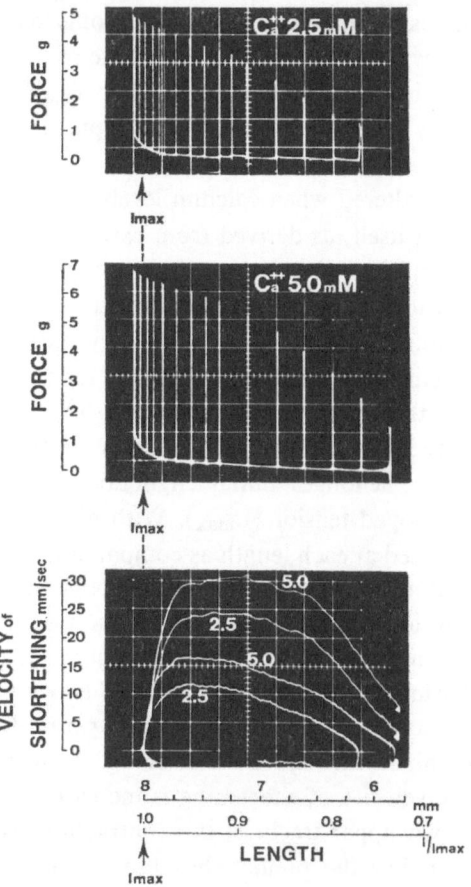

Fig. 7. Effects of unloading of a cat papillary muscle during shortening at two different calcium concentrations of 2.5 and 5.0 mM.
Upper and middle sections: Length-tension relations of the papillary muscle (same length scale as in upper 2 sections).
Lower section: velocity-length relationships for four isotonic contractions. In the upper two curves the preload of 0.7 g (L_max) was subtracted according to the resting length-tension relationships, while in the lower two curves the preload was maintained constant throughout shortening. Reproduced by permission from *Circulat. Res.*

remains constant, within 5% of its peak, over a range of lengths between L_{max} and 12.5% below L_{max}. Below this range, the measured velocity under unloaded conditions decreases with decreasing length. Similar observations were made for various other inotropic interventions. From these results it can be concluded that inotropic interventions greatly alter maximum velocity of shortening at all lengths, whereas changes in the initial muscle length certainly do not, at least not over the physiological range of lengths in functioning heart muscle.

Thus, applying these concepts to the intact heart, it seems that from a theoretical point of view V_{max} still represents a most valuable index of contractility. This index allows us to distinguish between the variations in the performance of the heart due to changes of the initial muscle length, and the variations caused by any inotropic intervention. However, a discussion of the limitations of the techniques, which are used for the application of these principles to the intact heart, does not fall within the scope of the present report and will be dealt with by the next speaker in this symposium.

REFERENCES

1. Henderson, A. H., Forman, R., Brutsaert, D. L. & Sonnenblick, E. H., Tetanic contraction in mamalian cardiac muscle. *Cardiovasc. Res.* Suppl. 1, 96-100 (1971).

2. Brady, A. J., Time and displacement dependence of cardiac contractility: problems in defining the active state and force-velocity relations. *Fed. Proc.* 24, 1410-1420 (1965).

3. Sonnenblick, E. H., Active state in heart muscle: its delayed onset and modification by inotropic agents. *J. gen. Physiol.* 50, 661-676 (1967).

4. Edman, K. A. P. & Nilsson, E., Mechanical parameters of myocardial contraction studies at a constant length of the contractile element. *Acta physiol. scand.* 72, 205-219, (1968).

5. Noble, M. I. M., Bowen, T. E. & Hefner, L. L., Force-velocity relationship of cat cardiac muscle, studied by isotonic and quick-release technique. *Circulat. Res.* 24, 821-833 (1969).

6. Brady, A. J., Are force and velocity parameters of cardiac contractility separable? (Abstract). *Cardiovasc. Res.* (Abstracts of the VI World Congress of Cardiology) p. 36. London 1970.

7. Brutsaert, D. L., Claes, V. A. & Sonnenblick, E. H., Effects of abrupt load alterations on force-velocity-length and time relations during isotonic contractions of heart muscle: load clamping. *J. Physiol.* (Lond.) 216, 319-330 (1970).

8. Ramsey, R. W. & Street, S. F., Isometric length-tension diagram of isolated skeletal muscle fibers of the frog. *J. cell. comp. Physiol.* 15, 11-34 (1940).

9. Gordon, A. M., Huxley, A. F. & Julian, F. J., The variation in isometric tension with sarcomere length in vertebrate muscle fibers. *J. Physiol.* (Lond.). 184, 170-192 (1966).

10. Huxley, H. E., The mechanism of muscular contraction. *Science* 164, 1356-1366 (1966).

11. Rüdel, R. & Taylor, S. R., Striated muscle fibers: facilitation of contraction at short lengths by caffeine. *Science* 172, 387-388 (1971).

12. Taylor, S. R. & Rüdel, R., Striated muscle fibers: Inactivation of contraction induced by shortening. *Science* 167, 882-884 (1970).

13. Huxley, A. F., Muscle structure and theories of contraction. *Prog. Biophys.* 7, 255-318 (1957).

14. Brutsaert, D. L., Claes, V. A. & Sonnenblick, E. H., Velocity of shortening of un-loaded heart muscle and the length-tension relation. *Circulat. Res.* 29, 63-75 (1971).

15. Civan. M. M. & Podolsky, R. J., Contraction kinetics of striated muscle fibres following quick changes in load. *J. Physiol.* (Lond.). 184, 511-534 (1966).

16. Armstrong, C. F., Huxley, A. F. & Julian, F. J., Oscillatory responses in frog skeletal muscle fibers. *J. Physiol.* (Lond.). 186, 26-27 P (1966).

17. Brutsaert, D. L., *Vergelijkende studie over de dubbele stimulatie-potentiering, de post-extrasystolische potentiering en de frequentiepotentiering van de contractiliteit van het hart.* Aggregation thesis. Gent 1967.

18. Brutsaert, D. L., Parmley, W. W. & Sonnenblick, E. H., Effects of various inotropic interventions on the dynamic properties of the contractile elements in heart muscle of the cat. *Circulat. Res.* 27, 513-522 (1970).

19. Brutsaert, D. L. & Sonnenblick, E. H., Nature of the force-velocity relation in heart muscle. *Cardiovasc. Res.* Suppl. 1, 18-33 (1971).

20. Sonnenblick, E. H., Implications of muscle mechanics in the heart. *Fed. Proc.* 21, 974-990 (1962).

21. Katz, A. M., Contractile proteins of the heart. *Physiol. Rev.* 50, 63-158 (1970).

22. Ebashi, S. & Endo, M., Calcium ion and muscle contraction. In: Butler, J. A. V. & Noble, D. (eds.), *Progress in biophysics and molecular biology*, pp. 123-183. Oxford 1968.

23. Brutsaert, D. L., Claes, V. A. and Goethals, M., *Effect of calcium on force-velocity-length relations of heart muscle of the cat.* Submitted for publication 1972.

QUANTITATIVE ASSESSMENT OF
LEFT VENTRICULAR FUNCTION

P. G. HUGENHOLTZ, G. T. MEESTER, B. S. TABAKIN AND J. HEIKKILÄ

A problem of continuing concern to the clinical cardiologist is the evaluation of myocardial muscle function apart from the performance of the ventricle as a pump. This is of special importance when surgical intervention to correct abnormal haemodynamic loads imposed by valvular lesions or abnormal shunt is considered. Due to various compensations in the event of heart failure, moderate to severe loss of myocardial function may not become manifest as ventricular pump failure until late in the course of disease, or unless the system is stressed. Alternatively, excessive flow or pressure loads may induce pump failure while the underlying myocardium is still relatively competent. Thus, the need to determine the function of the underlying myocardium independent of the load becomes essential. So far, a variety of indices derived from routine haemodynamic measurements has been utilized in an attempt to assess quantitatively the overall ventricular performance. However, most of these indices reflect only indirectly one or more of three separate but interdependent factors: (1) the intrinsic contractile state or contractility of the myocardium, (2) the end-diastolic volume or fiber length of the ventricle (preload), and (3) the impedance to ventricular ejection (afterload).

In view of the fact that the heart is a muscle with definable mechanical characteristics, recent studies have been directed toward the analysis of ventricular performance in terms of the underlying muscle properties. In several studies of animals the principles derived from isolated muscle mechanics have now been applied to the intact ventricle and these studies have demonstrated an inverse relationship between velocity of shortening and load in the functioning animal heart, in other words, the force-velocity relationship. Isolated muscle studies have shown that the maximal velocity of shortening at zero load (V_{max}) is characteristic of the contractile state of the muscle which is independent of initial muscle length. In man, however, such studies have generally been limited to the ejection phase of ventricular contraction when the relationships between force and velocity are more complex, since afterload and fiber length cannot be excluded from the calculations. In view of the studies in animals which have shown that V_{max} may be a sensitive measure of the contractile state of the heart, we felt that an attempt to obtain similar information in man would be of value.

In the present study, the relationship between contractile element velocity and stress has been derived from the isovolumetric portion of left ventricular contraction and V_{max} has been obtained both by a complex method which combines pressure measurement with quantitative angiography and by a simplified method which utilizes pressure measurements alone. It is the purpose of this analysis to show that determination of V_{max}, as an indicator of muscle performance, provides a sensitive and reproducible method for assessing myocardial contractility in man.

When focal areas of the cardiac muscle are infarcted the disrupted and uncoordinated left ventricular contraction leads to a less effective pump. Work is spent in changing shape rather than in the ejection of blood and thus may be termed 'wasteful' in lieu of 'useful' work. This difference becomes clinically obvious when a portion of the left ventricular wall remains non-contractile or when it balloons out during systole. Under such circumstances neither the 'total' ventricular performance studies nor the 'force-velocity' analyses are able to define whether the observed deterioration in function is due to a diffuse scarring of the muscle throughout the left ventricle – as found in widespread coronary artery disease – or to a combination of marked asynergy in circumscribed areas with a normal or even compensatory supernormal function of uninvolved regions. As modern surgical techniques have now made the resection of such non-functioning areas possible, quantitative methods to determine the relative contribution of a damaged and an uninvolved segment to the generation of the total left ventricular function need to be developed.

A decrease in myocardial contractile function is associated with a reduction in the extent and the velocity of myocardial fiber shortening. Therefore in this study, fiber shortening was first measured by means of radiopaque markers placed on various epicardial segments of the left ventricle before and after experimentally induced myocardial infarction. Secondly, similar measurements were carried out to determine the extent and velocity of changes in transmural wall thickness. In order to decide whether the change in left ventricular wall thickening was as informative as the extent of epicardial ventricular shortening, both were compared before and after myocardial infarction of the anterior wall and related to control measurements of the posterior wall. As radiopaque markers cannot be placed in clinical situation except after cardiac surgery, and wall thickness may be studied from single plane angiocardiograms, the method would have the advantage of permitting regional myocardial function analysis under clinical circumstances.

To evaluate the usefulness of V_{max} calculated on the basis of the Hill model for muscle, several approaches were tried. In the absence of a reliable clinical or haemodynamic reference standard (with the exception of the four patients who died since the study was started), the evaluation of any index of myocardial contractility is difficult in intact man. For example, indices of performance conventionally employed, and therefore included in this analysis, are themselves dependent on factors other than contractility and thus constitute a poor reference. Indeed this may form a major reason for some of the scatter observed (Fig. 1).

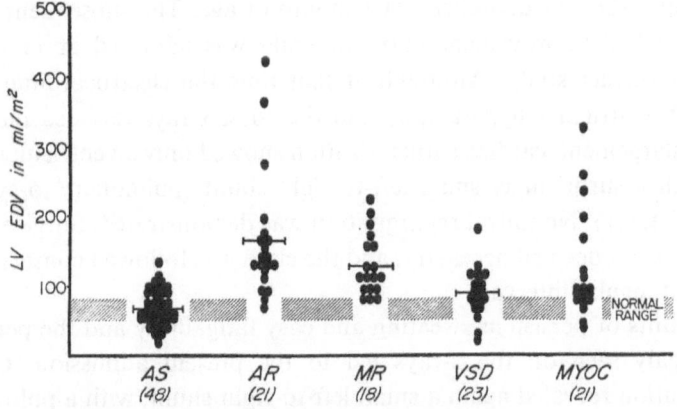

Fig. 1. Data on measured end-diastolic left ventricular volume in various diseases. Values are corrected for Body surface area.
AS: Aortic Stenosis
AR: Aortic Regurgitation
MR: Mitral Regurgitation
VSD: Ventricular Septal Defect
MYOC: Myocardiopathies

Nevertheless, the data show that at the ends of the spectrum, when all techniques agreed, V_{max} proved to be a good predictor of the clinical course. For example, patient J.S. was investigated at 16 months of age because of severe congestive heart failure. Catheterization revealed critical aortic stenosis with a peak gradient between left ventricle and aorta of 140 mm Hg.

However, the normal L VED P, L VEDV and E F, and the V_{max} of 4.9 circ/sec all suggest relatively good muscle function. This child had aortic valvulotomy, is now growing well and is completely asymptomatic 2 years after operation. On the other hand, the low V_{max} in J.F., a 17-year-old boy with equally severe signs of congestive heart failure clinically, portended a poor prognosis. Eight months after this study, autopsy showed severe subacute myocarditis. A total of five patients have died within a period of 4 to 9 months after cardiac catheterization. The values for V_{max} for these five were all below 2.5 circ/sec and the average for the group was 1.7 circ/sec.

It seemed of interest, however, to scrutinize that group of patients who had a low V_{max} without haemodynamic evidence of poor myocardial function. C.R., a 9-year-old child who developed difficulty in feeding when 2 weeks old and pneumonia 1 week later, is an example. Because of increased sweating, grossly increased heart size and other clear signs of congestive heart failure, she was digitalized at 1 month of age. The subsequent course showed gradual improvement until the child was admitted at 11 months of age for further study. Although at that time the electrocardiogram revealed left ventricular hypertrophy and the chest x-rays revealed moderate cardiac enlargement, cardiac catheterization showed only a ventricular septal defect with a surprisingly small left-to-right shunt (pulmonary-to-systemic flow ratio, 1.4:1). No mitral regurgitation was demonstrated. Surgical intervention was not deemed necessary, and the child was followed conservatively and seen at regular intervals.

Complaints of persistent sweating and easy fatigability and the persistent cardiomegaly seen on the x-rays led to the present admission. Cardiac catheterization revealed again a small left-to-right shunt, with a pulmonary-to-systemic flow ratio of only 1.1:1. The end-diastolic pressure and volume as well as the ejection fraction were within normal limits. In view of the abnormal V_{max} calculated over three consecutive beats, it is now believed that this child indeed has a subtle abnormality in myocardial function which was not demonstrated by conventional catheterization data. As a matter of fact, only the finding of a low V_{max} appears to explain the persistent cardiomegaly, the severe bout of congestive heart failure in infancy and the subtle signs of impaired myocardial function, which seem out of proportion to the demonstrated size of the ventricular septal defect and left-to-right shunt.

In another patient in this group, V_{max} appeared to show abnormalities of myocardial contractility without clear-cut evidence of abnormal function of the cardiac pump. C.M. is a 10-year-old girl who was asymptomatic. She was referred for evaluation because of a systolic murmur and an abnormal electrocardiogram. Although the L V E D P, L V E D V and E F were within normal limits, the E C G showed severe left ventricular hypertrophy with T-wave inversion, and the angiocardiogram revealed a greatly thickened left ventricular wall. No gradient could be demonstrated between the left ventricular cavity and aorta, even after the infusion of isoproterenol in large amounts. While the conventional haemodynamic data showed no abnormality in the cardiac pumping action, V_{max} was abnormally low. In keeping with the findings by Spann and co-workers, the low V_{max} would indicate poor myocardial contractility secondary to intrinsic muscle disease.

Three of the other patients in this group with low values had indirect evidence of impaired muscle function. L.M. is a 29-year-old woman with rheumatic mitral stenosis and regurgitation who may have a myocardial component to her rheumatic heart disease that has not yet shown any obvious haemodynamic abnormalities. Also, she is the oldest patient in the study; the effect of age on V_{max} has not been determined. M.Dr. was affected by a severe episode of acute rheumatic fever in early youth which left him with mild aortic valve insufficiency. S.C. had an atrial septal defect, and it is of some interest that patients with A S D have shown abnormal muscle function when challenged by isoproterenol. Thus, it may be suggested that some

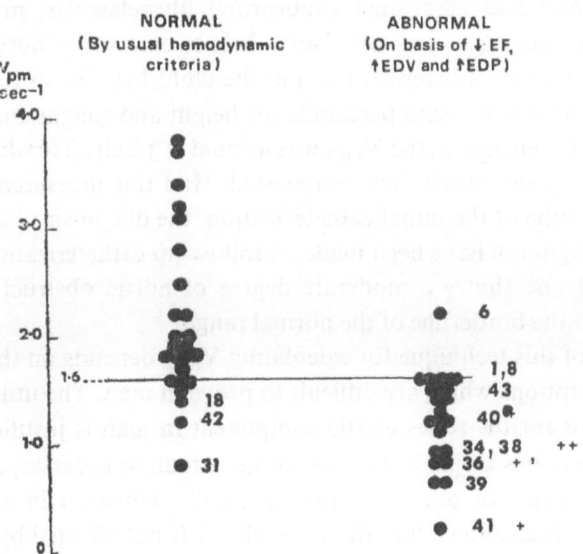

Fig. 2. Comparison of V_{max} with other parameters.
V_{max} calculated from left ventricular pressure is shown against classification on the basis of other haemodynamic criteria.

element of left ventricular dysfunction exists with pure right ventricular overloads, and this view warrants further study.

One other group of patients deserves notice. (Fig. 2). These are the patients in whom the pumping action of the heart appears impaired on the basis of an increased end-diastolic pressure or volume or a decreased ejection fraction, while the V_{max} suggests normal or only borderline depression of myocardial muscle function. One of the patients in this group RR, has aortic stenosis and his abnormal haemodynamic state may represent an increase in afterload rather than an impairment of muscle function. RA is a patient with idiopathic hypertrophic subaortic stenosis who was also believed to have an excessive afterload upon initial study. It is interesting that a second study, after treatment with large doses of the beta-adrenergic blocking agent propranolol for almost 2 years, showed that V_{max} had decreased. Whether this represents decreased muscle function due to progression of his muscle disease or suppression of function secondary to the propranolol itself is not known. Another interesting patient in this group is RO, a 3-year-old child who developed severe congestive heart failure at 1 month of age. Cardiac catheterization revealed critical aortic stenosis, and because of the greatly elevated L V E D P (to 33 mm Hg) and the decreased E F (0.47), it was felt that the child had associated endocardial fibroelastosis, making the indication for surgery questionable. Nevertheless, emergency aortic valvulotomy was done after catheterization, and the child has shown remarkable progress. He is now in the 50th percentile for height and weight and remains asymptomatic. In retrospect, the V_{max} was normal at 3.8 circ/sec which would suggest that adequate muscle function existed. Had this measurement been available at the time of the initial catheterization, the diagnosis of associated fibroelastosis might not have been made. A follow-up catheterization 3 years after the initial one shows a moderate degree of aortic obstruction while V_{max} remains at the borderline of the normal range.

Application of this technique for calculating V_{max} depends on the validity of several assumptions which are difficult to prove in man. The utilization of a single constant for the series elastic component in man is justified empirically. Further studies to prove this assumption remain necessary, particularly in hypertrophied or otherwise altered muscle. However in animal experiments, it has been shown that the series elastic is not affected by a variety of acute or chronic interventions or by either cardiac hypertrophy or failure provided a synchronous and symmetrical contraction is present. Since the data in this report were obtained for the most part from children, where segmental coronary heart disease is unlikely, the latter restriction appears not to have been violated.

Even so, the use of 28 as the constant in these calculations of series elasticity may eventually have to be revised. A second limitation lies in the fact that, while V_{max} was calculated under resting circumstances, heart rates did vary. Data published by Covell and co-workers show that V_{max} may increase as a function of heart rate. Both factors deserve further study; however, it is unlikely that they would materially affect the results of this study.

Another objection to be raised against the calculation of V_{max} is the extrapolation of the data over a significant distance to the hypothetical point of zero load. In isolated papillary muscle and intact animal experiments (at low EDP) this extrapolation appears to be justified. However, in man, this procedure may yield spurious results, especially in patients with high end-diastolic pressure and stress. Nevertheless, in this group of 35 studies, little qualitative difference was observed when extrapolation was performed to zero stress or zero developed stress. The entire question regarding the exact mode of extrapolation if any, particularly in instances of high end-diastolic stress, remains open to further investigation. Other objections that may be raised as to the validity of the haemodynamic data relate to the fact that in the majority of cases, pressure recordings were obtained by conventional fluid-filled catheters and transducer systems.

While potential distortion of pressure pulses by utilizing fluid-filled catheters rather than catheter-tip manometers is recognized, comparative studies in six instances in the present series did not alter the finding. However, subtle abnormalities of V_{max} and related values may be overlooked even with well-flushed catheters and for this reason, catheter-tip manometers appear advisable for use in future studies.

Also, a point must be made regarding the frequency of observation points during isovolumic contraction. While such points were obtained at 5-msec intervals after interpolation from a composite of films taken at random during several cycles, or at 8.3 msec when cineangiograms were used, real observations were still at least 16.7 sec apart with the cineangiograms, and frequently even further apart when the 6/sec biplanes were taken. Higher filming speeds which would increase the number of observation points to 10 or 12 during the isovolumic phase are much preferred. Studies involving these investigations are now in progress.

Balancing these objections is a solid base of evidence in animals that the technique does in fact meet the demands mentioned earlier for an index of contractility. V_{max} as calculated in these experiments has been shown to be independent of end-diastolic fiber length and systolic loading, and to be sensitively dependent on the inotropic state of the myocardial muscle. Despite the limitations of this technique when applied to man the present analysis suggests that V_{max} supplies information regarding myocardial contractility not otherwise available from data conventionally derived from cardiac catheterization.

It should also be noted that the use of ventricular angiography to define fiber motion as well as tension in the wall of the ventricle permits an estimation of V_{max} despite valvular regurgitation or interventricular shunting. Nevertheless, the simplified derivation utilizing pressure measurements alone appears adequate in most instances as indicated by the good correlation obtained between the two methods. This does not vitiate the need for ventriculography to exclude problems of valvular insufficiency, interventricular shunting and asynchronous ventricular contraction. In these latter situations more complex analyses may be required. In addition methods for obtaining V_{max} or similar indices will obviously undergo further refinement to improve ease of calculation and accuracy of measurement.

Further application of this technique to larger numbers of patients and to patients with different cardiac disorders will be required to validate the use of this parameter in the assessment of cardiac muscle function apart from the function of the entire heart as a pump. The significance of such measurements lies in the fact that they offer an opportunity to assess myocardial function in a quantitative fashion, such that abnormalities in contraction may be elicited prior to the manifestation of overt pump failure. Conversely, even in the presence of pump failure due to excessive loading, the adequacy of the muscle function per se may be assessed. It can be expected that such an analysis will permit a more rational approach to the advisability of surgical intervention.

The extent and rate of epicardial segment shortening and transmural wall thickening were also studied in various ventricular regions of the left ventricle by highspeed cineradiography of metal clips and by cineventriculography in 15 open-chested pigs. Normal systolic epicardial shortening and thickening averaged 15.8% and 31.7% respectively from the end-diastolic values. An unexpected degree of thickening of the left ventricular wall was observed in the isovolumetric phase, to a mean of 31.2% of total systolic thickening. Isoproterenol enhanced contraction mechanics significantly, again mostly during the isovolumetric phase.

Both epicardial segment length and wall thickness completely separated transmural infarction areas from adjacent or remote regions with normal muscle function (p < 0.0005). Ventricular asynergy occurred, and often reached its maximum extent, in the isovolumetric phase. Force-velocity analysis using V_{max} or dp/dt/Kp confirmed deterioration of total ventricular function after coronary artery ligation. Increased segment length in association with normal rate of contraction in the uninvolved muscle areas was observed. This indicated Frank-Starling compensation immediately after acute infarction. Thus a quantitative approach to the assessment of the severity and extent of myocardial infarction is now possible as well.

In fact, a comparison was made between the clip and angiographic methods for defining the inner boundary of the left ventricular wall to decide whether the changes in wall thickness determined by angiography would be as accurate as those found using the clip method. A close correlation was found throughout most of the cycle for delineation of the endocardial surface. During the last part of systole the angiographic definition was not always clear in all areas, and the values of wall thickness in end-systole often abruptly exceeded those obtained by the clip method. It has been clearly demonstrated that difficulties in angiocardiographic assessment of myocardial wall thickness occur only in the late systole. Since the changes in extent and velocity of thickening in impaired myocardial function occur in the isovolumetric phase of contraction and because maximum velocity of contraction of ejection takes place during the first half of systole, reliable measurements may be derived from angiograms. Further, the angiographic smoothness of the endocardium at the end-systolic phase in severe coronary artery disease or in akinetic areas will aid this analysis. This is clearly evident also in the present study.

The clinical application of the wall thickness analysis method in assessment of regional myocardial function is easily performed in many selected areas of the left ventricular wall, and even from single plane ventriculograms, as reported in two patients with coronary artery disease by Eber et al. This method may then provide an advantage of simplicity when compared with the elegant method of Kong et al. which assesses segmental myocardial function from spatial computations of biplane visualization of coronary artery motions.

The availability of analysis of regional function of the left ventricle combined with haemodynamic studies is of decisive importance in planning acute or elective surgical resection of an akinetic area after myocardial infarction. In these sometimes urgent situations it is difficult to assess whether critical deterioration of the circulation is due to extensive asynergic areas, or due to generalized diffuse scarring of the musculature. It is suggested that careful analysis of thickness changes of the left ventricular wall in the isovolumetric and ejection phases will provide the necessary insight.

In summary, this presentation emphasizes the degree to which quantitative measurements of left ventricular function may be made from biplane (or single plane) angiocardiography and illustrates its clinical significance to the cardioradiologist.

DISCUSSION

Sayers: The first two speakers hinted that there are some questions about the significance of the particular model used to represent the contractile element. Could you add anything to this?

Brutsaert: There is more and more agreement among the different workers that no one model is entirely suitable. Much of the controversy in myocardial contractility deals indeed with the model employed. The starting point for our unloading experiment was a model experiment; there we unloaded the muscle according to the length-tension relationship. Such instantaneous unloading is based upon the Maxwell model in which the contractile elements are clamped during shortening. However, if one considers a two-component model, one does not obtain direct information about the contractile elements during this type of unloading. Indeed, one could ask the question what would happen if the muscles were unloaded not according to the length-tension relationship, but according to other functions. Therefore, in addition to the controlled unloadings, we performed experiments with 'zero load clampings' in which the muscle was suddenly unloaded after the latent period, i.e. clamping the load from the preload to zero load.

After an initial transient, the curve followed the same phase-plane relationship as during unloading according to the length-tension relationship. We then performed unloadings between the two extremes and all of the curves showed an initial transient before returning to the same phase plane. In view of this, one can indeed question the need for utilizing other models. With a simple two-component model one would obtain similar results. Thus, all of the arguments about which model to use in heart muscle are rather unimportant except for the first portion of the contraction prior to the peak velocity value. It is also important in the transition from the resting condition to an active condition. Likewise in the intact heart the discussion of a model in plain contraction cycles is rather irrelevant.

Sandler: Dr. Hugenholtz proposed that we go along with Dr. Brutsaert in using the muscle physiology from isolated muscle for intact hearts. Where does he think he is going to get the evidence for really being able to apply isolated muscle findings to the intact heart? There is a lot to say hydraulic-ally, because there you really are looking at the integrated function of the muscle. Does he have any real evidence that we will be able to apply the isolated muscle data to the intact heart?

Hugenholtz: There are two comments that I would like to make. First of all that I concur with Dr. Brutsaert regarding the (ir)relevancy of models. At the extreme of the range of activity, i.e. excessive preload or afterload beyond the physiological range, no one model will necessarily apply to both condi-tions. However, in the physiologic range of the average patient, as far as we can make out, all models will fit. I am far more worried by problems such as the asynchrony in coronary heart disease. This is a very disturbing pro-blem and I would approach this area empirically.

Second, Dr. Sandler wants us to prove the 2nd Koch's postulate in the field as clinicians; in this context I would refer to the work that Meyler wants to do. That is to take the papillary muscle of the patient for whom he has the preoperative data and then to experiment on the isolated paipllary muscle from that particular individual. By comparing the data from angiocardio-grams while the heart was intact with the isolated muscle strip we should find the true relationships. This is a tremendous job but it could yield the proof of the postulate which you and I seek.

In the meantime, we are all living with a number of things which are in-completely understood and yet we use them. I am not going to wait until someone proves ultimately that these things are indeed related when in the meantime I can use these parameters in the catheterization laboratory now for the assessment of left ventricular muscle function as opposed to pump function.

Sandler: I see no evidence anywhere in the literature that there is any way we can separate hydraulic from muscle function. They are totally and completely in equilibrium. It is a matter of your frame of reference. You might look at the fluid being pumped, but it cannot be pumped unless the muscle acts in some way upon the fluid.

Hugenholtz: We have no disagreement there, but we have found examples of patients whose heart behaves properly as a pump but where the muscle is almost gone. What really has happened there is that preload and afterload have compensated to such an extent that the overall impression of the hydraulic evaluation is reasonable, whereas the muscle is bad. We have also had the opposite. Children, for instance, can be in gross failure (for example in aortic stenosis) and yet they have a very reasonable muscle function. What we are trying to say is that in the majority of cases, our assessment of pump function will be enough. However, there will be circumstances when we will be unable to determine if a patient has compensated and, if so, under what conditions. If you really want to get at this in a more exact way you will have to separate the three components: those related to preload, those to afterload and those to specific muscle function e.g. 'contractility'.

Selvester: I have a question for Dr. Tabakin. I think experience has shown that we come right up to the edge of disaster before hydraulic measurements indicate failure. The homeostatic mechanisms compensate so completely that we get to the very edge before we fall over. Could you comment from your data or others how close to that brink we really go.

Tabakin: Obviously we don't know the answer to that yet. It is one of the things we are looking for. I think that one must continue to take measurements and set up correlations. The haemodynamic measurements are difficult to have continuously on-line. Those of us who have worked in exercise studies and dye-dilution are aware of the tremendous variation that you can have in cardiac output from minute to minute. You can measure cardiac output with a dye dilution curve in the coronary care unit and two hours later it may no longer represent anything like the actual cardiac output. We must have some way of following it continuously. That is what we are looking for and that is what Dr. Hugenholtz was pointing out about the fiberoptic or thermal dilution curves because they may be *the* way of getting at the problem. We have some evidence now to believe that the systolic time intervals may be extremely helpful in this and perhaps we can include them in the program. I do not think that anyone knows when the patient is at the brink and when we should jump in. This is a decision we face daily not only in the coronary care unit, but also in the clinical situation when we are catheterizing our patients and we try to avoid a mortality during the procedure. We do not know the exact point of intervention.

Sandler: We were all taught that we should measure the patient at rest and from that measurement we would obtain all of the information that was necessary to make our predictions. We now know we must do some provocative tests. As Dr. Hugenholtz indicated, you can use pacing, exercise or

Isuprel. That is the only way to gauge how close to the edge you are. To take a measurement solely and completely at rest of a physiologic system which has a vast reserve capacity is very misleading and even dangerous. When applied to clinical patients you will never know where you are in the natural course of a disease process if you use such an approach.

Sayers: I am sure that there is no argument about this at all. We are at a point where dynamic response measurements are absolutely crucial. The behavior of a system which does have the ability of compensating for the failure or partial failure of some of its elements is very complicated. You can't stand and look at it without running the risk of falling over the edge before you know you are there. This is a characteristic that any engineer would recognize in a feed-back system. Any such system, whether it is a simple one or very complex, behaves very well indeed until it is pushed beyond its limits and then it collapses catastrophically.

Selvester: Dr. Hemker's notions, yesterday, intrigued me a great deal. It seems to me that if we can solve the problem of how much myocardium we have lost, we'll have some indication of how close to that brink we are. It is pretty well established now that that brink does not occur until a large amount of myocardium has been destroyed. Some people say 35 and some say 50 percent. It is somewhere in that range.

LEFT VENTRICULAR SIZE AND FUNCTION

METHODS FOR THE ANALYSIS OF
ANGIOCARDIOGRAPHIC DATA*

P. H. HEINTZEN, P. E. LANGE, V. MALERCZYK AND J. PILARCZYK

Angiocardiography is the visual documentation of the spatial distribution and the temporal changes of x-ray absorption caused by contrast-filled cardiovascular structures.

The quantitative analysis of this graphic information is called angiocardiometry.

Roentgendensitometry means transformation of x-ray absorption or roentgendensity into an optical correlate and particularily its conversion into an electrical signal, which can be recorded by adequate photoelectrical transducers (photomultipliers, flying spot scanners or television cameras). (1)

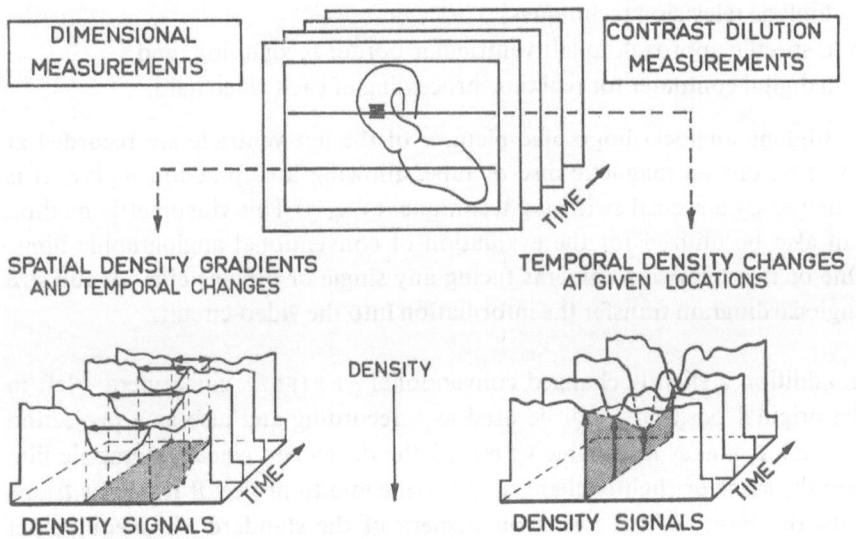

Fig. 1. The two main ways to quantitate angiocardiographic data by different analyses of density signals.

* Supported by the Volkswagen Foundation.

The two main ways to quantitate angiocardiographic data are based on the different analyses of the density signals (Fig. 1):

– One determines the dimensions by utilizing local densities and spatial density gradients.

– The other applies the indicator dilution principle to radiopaque material, recording the temporal density changes and gradients at a given site.

Descriptions follow of the methods available for:

1. automated videometric or cine-videometric measurements of cardiovascular dimensions, especially left ventricular volume;
2. synchronization of angiocardiographic data with various reference signals;
3. automated documentation of angiocardiograms to get a complete protocol of heart catheterization data, and
4. the application of the indicator dilution principle to cine- and videoangiograms.

1. Our method for automated volume determination of cardiovascular structures (2) uses:
a. biplane television techniques;
b. a specific approach to left ventricular border recognition, and
c. a digital computer for real time processing of each video field.

a. Biplane angiocardiographic pictures of the left ventricle are recorded at 50 or 60 cps on magnetic disc or tape, allowing a stop action replay. It is achieved by a special switching technique. (3, 4, 5) This videometric method can also be utilized for the evaluation of conventional angiographic films. One or two television cameras facing any single or biplane cine- or full size angiocardiogram transfer the information into the video-circuit.

In addition a slightly changed conventional ARRIFLEX cinecamera – left in the original position – can be used as a recording and also as a projection device.* It makes it possible to reload the developed cineangiographic film into the same or slightly changed magazine and to project it frame by frame onto the target of the television camera of the standard x-ray equipment without the need for any additional projector, videocamera or optical system (Fig. 2). In each case a videographic display is the input information for the next step of the procedure.

---

* Pat. pending.

b. On the basis of our experience with clinical and experimental angiocardiography and extensive studies of density signals from the heart with and without contrast media we came to the conclusion that at the present time there is no realistic chance for a completely automated method for heart

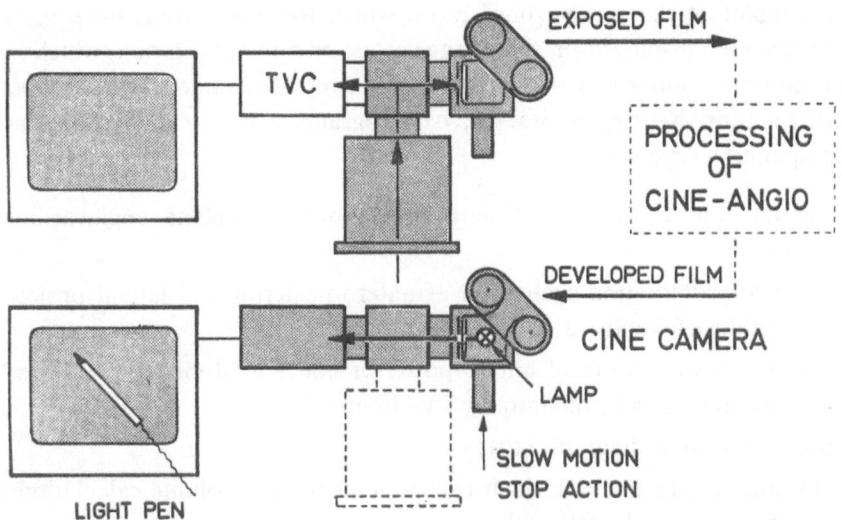

Fig. 2. Slightly changed conventional ARRIFLEX cinecamera (lower section), which allows the utilization of standard heart catheterization equipment for videometric evaluation of developed cineangiocardiograms. (TVC = television camera).

border recognition. Therefore the heart borders are defined by an experienced cardiologist. To do this we use a light pen (6) to trace the cardiac silhouette of each individual frame. These drawn cardiac borders (and the pressure values) are stored for control and further processing by inscribing the contours onto the screen of a storage oscilloscope, scan converter or digital matrix.

c. The stored border information can than be read out for computer analysis either by facing a videocamera against the storage scope (7), by switching the scan converter into the 'read' mode, or – as has become possible recently – by operating the scanner in the 'read/write' mode.

Each scanning videoline crossing the heart borders or pressure marks is characterized by 2 to 4 bright border pulses. These pulses are coded and used to start and stop 4 digital counters in such a way that the counter content is proportional to the time difference between the border pulses and thus to the distance between the cardiac borders. The counters are buffered and read into the computer every 64 μs via a 32 bit direct digital input. Starting with an interrupt, derived from the vertical sync pulse, each video field is read into the computer line per line in real time. The digital computer identifies the information and calculates the actual volume. The results and a replot of the cardiac borders on which the calculations have been based are then displayed on the storage scope of a remote station, which is built into our volume console. Executed and controlled under the CDC 1700 MEDLAB time-sharing monitor (8, 9), programs can be called from the corresponding keyboard for:

a. simultaneous evaluation of both projections of biplane angiocardiograms;

b. successive alternating evaluation of antero-posterior and lateral projections of the left ventricle;

c. subsequent evaluation of antero-posterior and lateral cine-angiocardiographic films, transferred into the TV-circuit;

d. pressure-volume diagrams (10);

e. videometric planimetry, which can be used for the volume calculations based on the area-length method.

In addition a series of 'Off Line' programs is available for calculation of other commonly used parameters.

For programs 1 to 4, a so-called 'blow up' procedure (2) is utilized (Fig. 3). If, for example, the lateral projection of the left ventricle is smaller than the corresponding antero-posterior one, the smaller silhouette is blown up in such a way that it has the same height or number of videolines as the antero-posterior counterpart. By interpolating, the length of the now larger number of axes is calculated and then corrected according to the horizontal scaling factors of the lateral plane. The accuracy of this method has been tested by using different models and comparing the results obtained at the in- and output of the disc recorder, after introducing the light pen, and finally at the output from the computer. (11, 12, 13) All correlation coefficients were higher than .99. For the standard sphere with a known volume of 113.04 ml the standard error of estimate was 2.5 ml, the standard error of the mean .25 ml and the percentage error of the mean value from these 100 determinations .06%. Systematic studies of dye-filled pig hearts and of plastic casts from these ventricles have demonstrated that the 'end-diastolic' volume can be determined with an error of ± 5 to 10%. (14, 15)

Fig. 2. Real-time syndromization of pathobiological data which ... with what ...

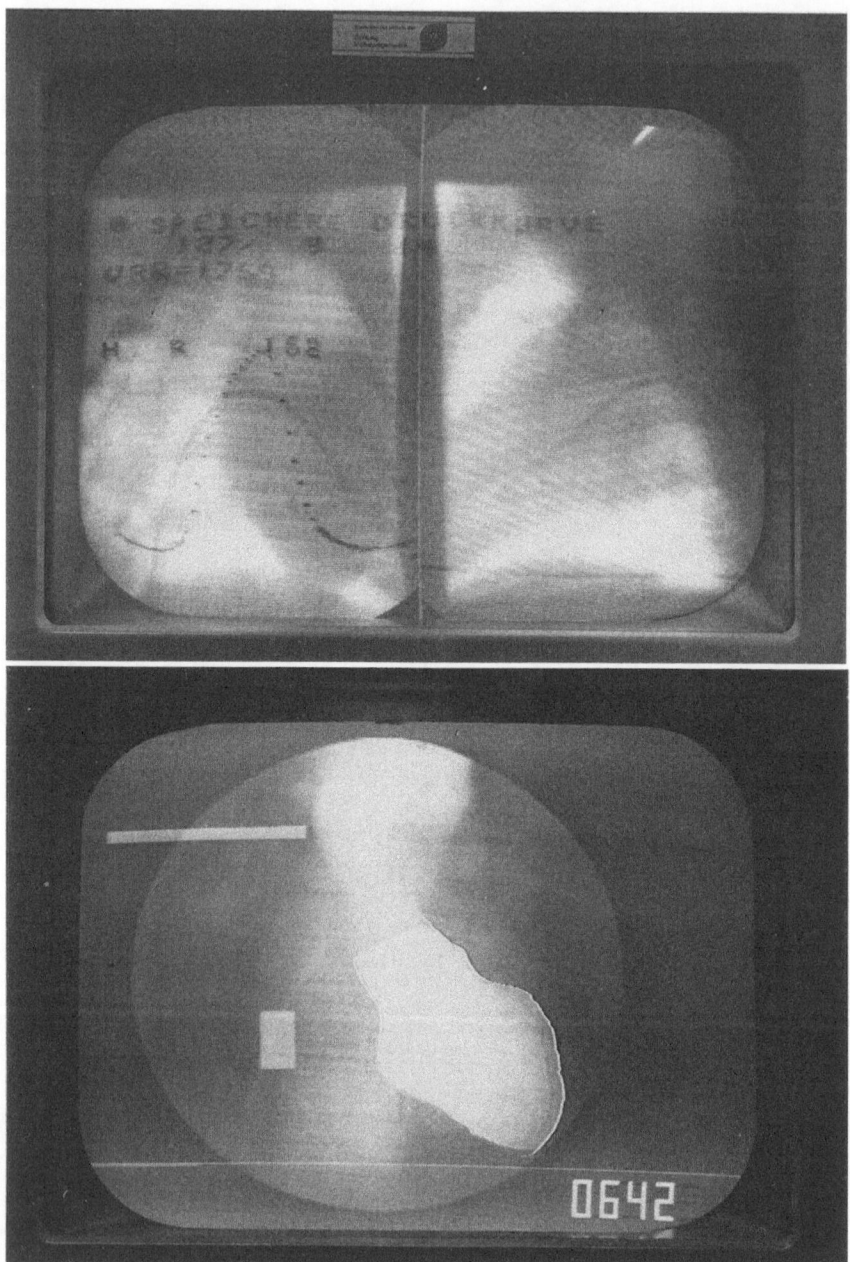

Fig. 4. Real time synchronization of morphological information with other reference values.

Upper section: biplane left ventricular angiocardiogram with fed in reference signals (like heart frequency, left ventricular pressure curve, etc.) from a storage oscilloscope of a remote computer station.

Lower section: left ventricular angiocardiogram with a pressure controlled video window (above), a standard rectangular video window and a contoured window outlining the left ventricle (middle), and the frame number (below).

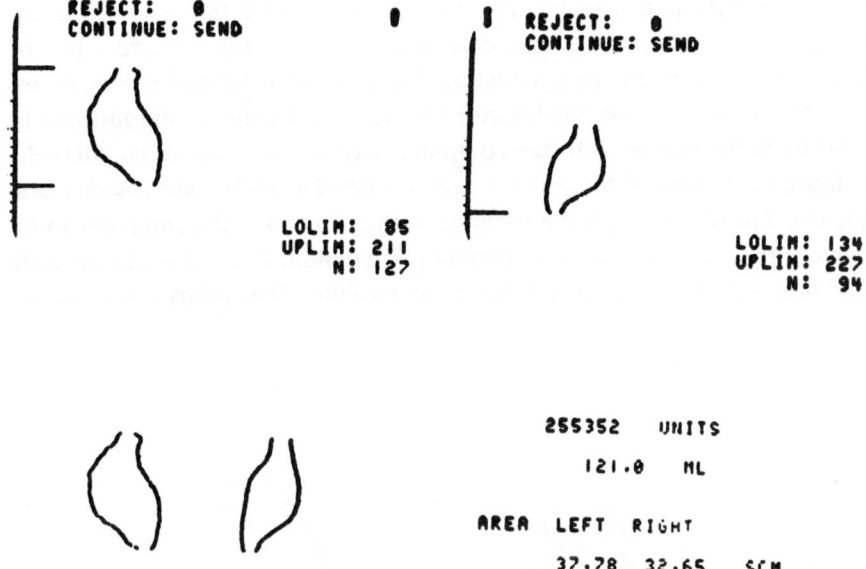

Fig. 3. 'Blow up' procedure, utilized for automated left ventricular volume determinations. (Displays on the scope of a scan converter-Tektronix 4501).
Left upper section: contour of traced left ventricular border in the ap projection.
Right upper section: contour of traced left ventricular border in the lateral projection.
Left lower section: contours of the traced left ventricular borders in the ap and the lateral projections. The originally smaller contour in the lateral projection (right upper section) is 'blown up', so that it now has the same number of videolines as the ap counterpart.
Right lower section: display of calculated left ventricular volume (above) and areas of the ap and lateral projections (below).

2. Real time synchronization of the morphological information with other physiological events or any other reference value in analog or digital form, such as patient identification, pressures, oxygen-saturation, etc. is possible too (Fig. 4). This can be achieved with a third TV-camera, which faces either an analog monitor or a storage oscilloscope of a remote computer station (16). At the present time however we use a scan converter to transmit all analog data from the computer directly into the biplane video picture. Character generators – now commercially available – enable us to feed into selected videolines digital numbers and characters of nearly all sizes and combinations (10, 17). For automated pressure/volume diagrams (10), for instance, instantenous pressures are transformed into voltages, which control the length of a bright horizontally moving 'electronic window', similar to those used in videodensitometry. Since pressure is visually included in the

video image it can be processed at the same time and in the same way as the morphological data for volume determination – described above – just by indicating the pressure, ECG, or calibration window by vertical marks, drawn with the light pen. Both the inscribed pressure and volume contours can be read from the scanner into the computer with the same set of counters developed for volume determination and described as *coding and counting unit* (2, 10). The difference in the program is that it enables the computer to recognize the counter content of certain predetermined videolines as pressure and others for instance, as, left ventricular volume. The information of each

SYSTOLE + DIASTOLE
AP

LATERAL

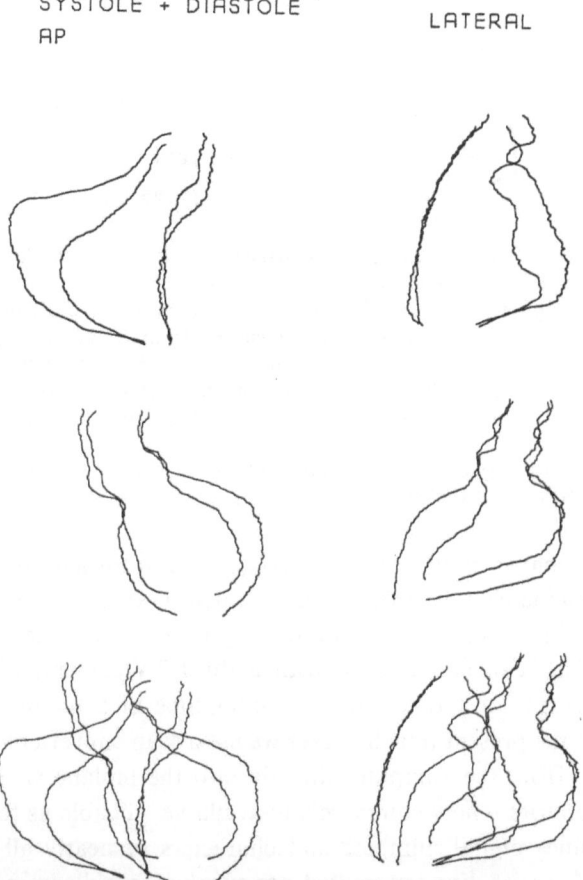

Fig. 5. Plotted end-systolic and end-diastolic contours in the ap (left) and lateral (right) projection of the right ventricle (above), the left ventricle (middle) and a superposition of both (below).

videoline is stored for further evaluation and can be displayed, for example, as pressure/volume diagrams.

3. Having a system of automated heart catheterization procedures (9) which gives us a protocol of all physiological data, comments and the relevant waveforms, we nevertheless missed the typical morphological or angiocardiographic information on the final hard-copy. Therefore we decided to extend our system in such a way that immediately following heart catheterization either an isodensity plot can be generated automatically from a selected videotape recording, or the typical shape of one or more cardiovascular structures (for instance the left ventricular cavity) can be drawn with a light pen. The data thus gained can be stored and printed or plotted out (Fig. 5, 6)

AP   LATERAL

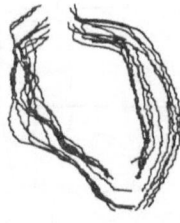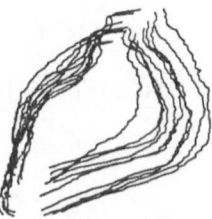

Fig. 6. Superposition of selected left ventricular, ap (left) and lateral (right), contours from one complete heart cycle.

(18). We expect this to be a practical and useful addition to the daily clinical routine.

The second main way to quantitate angiographic data is the application of the indicator dilution technique to conventional radiopaque material. To achieve this, three methods are available (Fig. 7):

1. The direct continuous recording of the temporal density changes from the fluorescent screen or the output phophor of an image intensifier;
2. Cinedensitometry, that is the density measurement within the cone of projection of an angiographic film;
3. Videodensitometry, that is the recording of the density changes by means of a TV-camera from which the specific video signals to be analysed are selected or gated out by a video window generator.

The latter technique – originally developed by Sturm, Sanders, and Wood in the Mayo Clinic (19) – has been improved during the last two years in our laboratory by:

a. making it applicable to clinical angiocardiography with pulsed radiation (20, 21, 22);

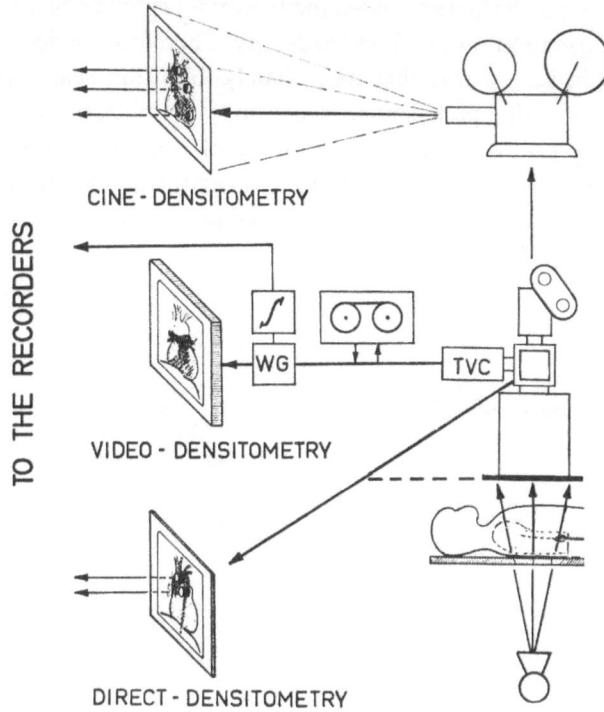

Fig. 7. Three methods available to quantitate angiocardiographic data by applying the indicator dilution principle to conventional radiopaque material. (WG = window generator, TVC = television camera).

b. allowing quantitative density measurements, by converting the original video signal logarithmically, and

c. by generating variable contoured video windows of any shape desired (23, 24).

This means that the two main ways to quantitate angiographic data merge. The contour storage capabilities are utilized to shape the video window as desired, thereby selecting the area from which density measurements are wanted.

Compared with conventional indicator dilution techniques roentgendensitometry of contrast material has the following important advantages:

1. indirect sampling is possible at nearly all sites of the circulation without the need of introducing special catheters for withdrawal of the indicator;
2. only one injection is required for any number of analyses, since the complete 'image' of the indicator passage is stored on magnetic tape, disc, or film for repeated evaluation and recording of density changes;
3. the amount of indicator can be measured at any desired area or simultaneously at different sites;
4. the dynamic response is fast, thus allowing the analysis of cyclic density changes from beat to beat (25, 26).

Since the basic requirements for quantitative density measurements – with respect to x-ray equipment, the laws governing x-ray absorption by contrast material and the recording system – have been fullfilled (20), roentgendensitometry has reached the stage of development where it can be transferred into the experimental and clinical laboratory as a safe and promising tool.

REFERENCES

1. Heintzen, P. H., (ed.), *Roentgen-, cine- and videodensitometry.* Stuttgart 1971.
2. Heintzen, P. H., Malerczyk, V., Pilarczyk, J. & Scheel, K. W., On-line processing of the video-image for left ventricular volume determination. *Computers and biomedical research* 4, 474 (1971).
3. Williams, J. C. P., Sturm, R. E., Tsakiris, A. G. & Wood, E. H. Biplane videoangiography. *J. appl. Physiol.* 24, 724 (1968).
4. Heintzen, P. H., Osypka, P. & Bürsch, J., New techniques for functional studies in radiology and cardiology. *Ann. Radiol.* 12, 425 (1969).
5. Osypka, P. & Heintzen, P. H., New applications of television techniques for quantitative measurements in radiology and cardiology. *Proc. 7th Conf. Med. Biol. Electronics* 108-110, Stockholm 1967.
6. Piltz, F. & Schafer, H., Fotoelektrischer Zeigestab für Fernsehbilder. *Radio-Mentor* 12, 938 (1964).
7. Heintzen, P. H., Moderne diagnostische Methoden in der Kardiologie. *Thoraxchirurgie* 18, 290 (1970).
8. Pryor, T. A. & Warner, H. R., Time sharing in biomedical research. *Datamation* 54 (1966).
9. Gardner, R. M., Pryor, T. A., Malerczyk, V. Pilarczyk, J. & Heintzen, P. H., Automatisierung der Herzkathetertechnik. *Z. Kreisl.-Forsch.* 59, 347 (1970).
10. Heintzen, P. H., Malerczyk, V. & Pilarczyk, J., A videometric technique for automated processing of pressure-volume diagrams. *Computers and biomedical research* 4, 486 (1971).
11. Heintzen, P. H., Malerczyk, V., Pilarczyk, J., Schohl, H. H. & Vogel G. W., Automa-

tisierung der röntgenologischen Herzkammervolumenbestimmung unter Einsatz eines magnetischen Bildplattenspeichers. *Röfo* 114, 215 (1971).

12. Schohl, H. H., *Röntgenvideometrische Bestimmung von Modellvolumina als Grundlage eines Verfahrens zur automatisierten Messung des Herzkammervolumens.* Thesis, Kiel 1971.

13. Vogel, G. W., *Möglichkeiten und Fehler einer automatisierten Volumenbestimmung aus Röntgenfernsehsignalen an Modellen.* Thesis, Kiel 1971.

14. Blauert, U., *Die Genauigkeit eines röntgenvideodensitometrischen Verfahrens zur Bestimmung des linksventrikulären Volumens, geprüft an Ausgußpräparaten von Schweineherzen.* Thesis, Kiel 1971.

15. Thies, J., *Die Genauigkeit eines röntgenvideodensitometrischen Verfahrens zur Bestimmung des linksventrikulären Volumens, geprüft an kontrastmittelgefüllten Schweineherzen.* Thesis, Kiel 1971.

16. Osypka, P., New techniques for processing medical videosignals and handling of reference data on videodisc recording. In: Heintzen, P. H. (ed.), *Roentgen-, cine- and videodensitometry.* p. 61. Stuttgart 1971.

17. Heintzen, P. H. & Pilarczyk, J., Videodensitometry with contoured and controlled windows. In: Heintzen, P. H. (ed.), *Roentgen-, cine- and videodensitometry.* p. 56. Stuttgart 1971.

18. Heintzen, P. H., Malerczyk, V. & Pilarczyk, J., Stand der Automatisierung der Herzkathetertechnik und der Angiographie. *Röfo Beiheft* 1971 (In press).

19. Sturm, R. E., Sanders, J. J. & Wood, E. H., A roentgen videodensitometer for circulatory studies. *Fed. Proc.* 23, 303 (1964).

20. Heintzen, P. H., Usefulness and limitation of conventional X-ray equipment for roentgendensitometric studies. In: Heintzen, P. H. (ed.), *Roentgen-, cine- and videodensitometry.* p. 1. Stuttgart 1971.

21. Heintzen, P. H., Videodensitometry with pulsed radiation. In: Heintzen, P. H. (ed.), *Roentgen-, cine- and videodensitometry.* p. 46. Stuttgart 1971.

22. Heintzen, P. H. & Moldenhauer, K., X-ray absorption by contrast material using pulsed radiation. In: Heintzen, P. H. (ed.), *Roentgen, cine- and videodensitometry.* p. 85. Stuttgart 1971.

23. Heintzen, P. H. & Moldenhauer, K., The x-ray absorption by contrast material. In: Heintzen, P. H. (ed.), *Roentgen- cine- and videodensitometry.* p. 73. Stuttgart 1971.

24. Bürsch, J., Johs, R., Kirbach, H., Schnürer, C. & Heintzen, P. H., Accuracy of videodensitometric flow measurement. In: Heintzen P. H. (ed.), *Roentgen-, cine- and videodensitometry.* p. 119. Stuttgart 1971.

25. Williams, J. C. P. & Wood, E. H., Application of roentgen videodensitometry to the study of mitral valve function. In: Heintzen, P. H. (ed.), *Roentgen-, cine- and videodensitometry.* p. 89. Stuttgart 1971.

26. Bürsch, J. & Heintzen, P. H., Messungen der Blutströmung und des Herzkammervolumens nach dem Prinzip der Indikatorverdünnungstechnik mittels Videodensitometrie. Presented at Congressus Secundus Societatis Radiologicae Europaeae, Amsterdam, June 14-18, 1971. (In press).

LEFT VENTRICULAR VOLUME, MASS AND RELATED MEASURES; USEFULNESS IN DETERMINATION OF VENTRICULAR FUNCTION

H. SANDLER

One of the most significant advances in the area of assessing cardiac performance over the past 20 years has been the ability to determine dimensions for isolated cardiac muscle or the intact heart. Dimensions and/or change in dimensions compared with simultaneously measured force or pressure have resulted in the now well-known length-tension and force velocity concepts and the ability to characterize the intact heart as a muscle or as a pump (1-6). The ability to measure dimensions in the intact heart, particularly in man, presents many unique problems. These include the need to use clinically acceptable methods for obtaining such information and to account for the complex configuration of the ventricular chambers. Figure 1 lists the various

A. DIRECT
BING CATHETER
RESISTANCE

B. INDIRECT
1. ULTRASONIC ECHO
2. X-RAY
   SINGLE PLANE
   BIPLANE
   EKY
   RADARKYMOGRAPHY
3. CLIPS
4. RADIOACTIVITY
5. INDICATOR DILUTION
   GREEN DYE
   HOT, COLD SALINE
   FIBEROPTIC

Fig. 1. Various methods for determining ventricular dimensions in man.

methods used for such purposes in man. These methods have varied from the use of special catheters (7) to strain gages or clips placed in the epicardial surface of the heart at surgery (8, 9) to the use of radioactive materials (10). X-ray methods have proven by far to be the most reliable methods for measuring cardiac chamber size and shape. Differences still exist among various investigators concerning the accuracy of x-ray and indicator dilution methods for measuring ventricular volume or size (11-14). Time is demonstrating that neither method is completely correct. Indicator dilution methods tend to overestimate end-diastolic volume (EDV); angiographic methods tend to overestimate the ejection fraction (EF). With careful concern for technique, these faults can be corrected in each system.

Ventricular dimensions are obtained from the x-ray films by measurement of chamber size and shape during angiocardiography as shown in figure 2.

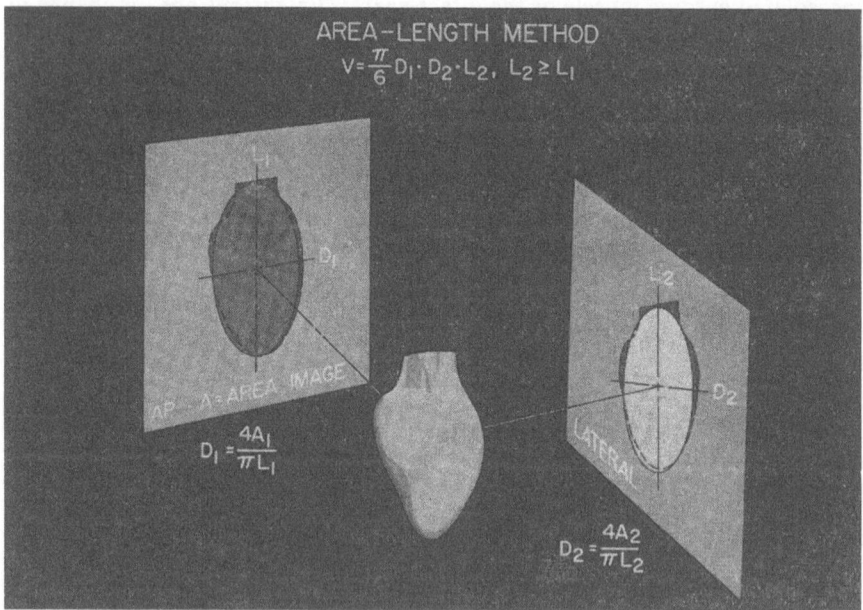

Fig. 2. Angiographic determination of ventricular size (area-length method).

The opacified left ventricular (LV) chamber, whether recorded on large films or by motion picture techniques, is assumed to represent a regular geometric figure, usually an ellipsoid (15). Chamber dimensions are directly measured or derived from the recorded images as shown. Volumes calculated by these methods are corrected or adjusted by statistical equations for overestimation of actual ventricular volumes (16). When such corrections are not used, the resulting errors are so large as to make calculated volumes unreliable. Measurement of lateral wall thickness allows for the determination of the volume of the shell representing L V muscle and allows for the calculation of L V mass (17). This latter method is the only means at present for determining L V mass in human subjects during life.

By using the above methods, ventricular size and shape can be determined for the several heart beats of chamber opacification during angiocardiography and correlated with simultaneously recorded heart rate and L V pressure. One of the first applications of this approach was a comparison of associated L V E D V and L V end-diastolic pressure (E D P) (18). It was demonstrated, contrary to assumptions prevalent at that time, that L V E D P and E D V were not linearily related for subjects with chronic heart disease of varied etiologies. Normal volume by angiocardiographic methods was determined to be between 75 to 125 ml. Many subjects with L V E D V 2, 3 or 4 times normal were demonstrated to have a normal L V E D P of 10 to 12 mm Hg.

The next application of dimensions for the study of cardiac function was a comparison of volume with simultaneously recorded pressure throughout the cardiac cycle. Such comparisons produced so-called pressure-volume (P-V) loops, the area enclosed within such loops representing the net work the L V performs in ejecting its stroke volume (S V) (5, 6). A comparison of P-V loops for various disease states demonstrated such procedures to be useful but not unique in characterizing performance (6). Normal values for stroke work were shown to be 45-65 G_m-M. Subjects with combined aortic stenosis and insufficiency were demonstrated to have the highest work requirements with values 8 to 10 times normal. Many subjects with pure aortic stenosis had values similar to subjects with mixed mitral valvular disease, the work being performed in an entirely different fashion in these respective cases. Many subjects with large hearts due to coronary artery disease or primary muscle disease had effective stroke work values which were normal, yet L V E D V was four times normal. Work values in such cases did not help differentiate the hydraulic defects in these latter cases. Several investigators have attempted to convert derived work values into power, since power represents the rate of doing work. Such calculations have helped somewhat to show differences in work capacity in such situations but have not clearly differentiated among various disease states (19).

Volume has been used alone to gage performance. The difference between E D V and end-systolic volume (E S V) represents the L V stroke volume (S V). L V S V must equal forward flow in the absence of valvular insufficiency when determined by some independent technique such as the Fick or indicator dilution method (6). In the presence of valvular insufficiency the difference between L V S V and forward flow must quantitatively measure the amount of regurgitation per beat. The ratio L V S V to E D V or the Ej F has also been shown to be a useful means of gaging performance. Subjects with myocardial disease have been shown to have low Ej F (6).

Chamber dimensions have proven to be extremely important in themselves. Derived values for change in size have been used to obtain the rate of ejection (20) or the overall percentage change of length or diameter from its respective end-diastolic value. Percentage change in diameter (equivalent to rate of circumferential fiber shortening) has recently been demonstrated to be linearly related to the Ej F as illustrated in figure 3. These studies have

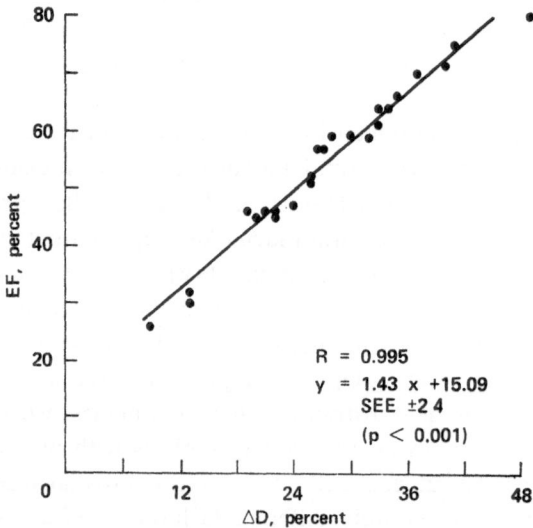

Fig. 3. Relationship between percentage change in diameter (%ΔD) and the ejection fraction (EF).

clearly shown that it is no longer necessary to record the entire cardiac silhouette in order to determine an Ej F. Such findings have direct applications to measurements made by newer methods such as cardiac echo ultrasound where L V diameter and change in diameter are usually the only parameters that can easily be derived (21). By using such methods, it is now possible to measure an Ej F based on these findings without using x-ray or other invasive procedures.

The ability to determine mass has helped determine function in patients with valvular or coronary artery disease (22, 23). Normal values for LV mass are below 200 Gm. Markedly increased masses have also been shown to be present in conditions such as aortic stenosis, primary myocardial disease and subaortic stenosis. It is now clear that work or performance should be gaged against the total mass of muscle present rather than simply by stroke volume, pressure or power alone.

The method for calculating volumes illustrated in figure 2 is used primarily for procedures which require information concerning ventricular size. Figure 4 demonstrates the method used for conditions requiring information con-

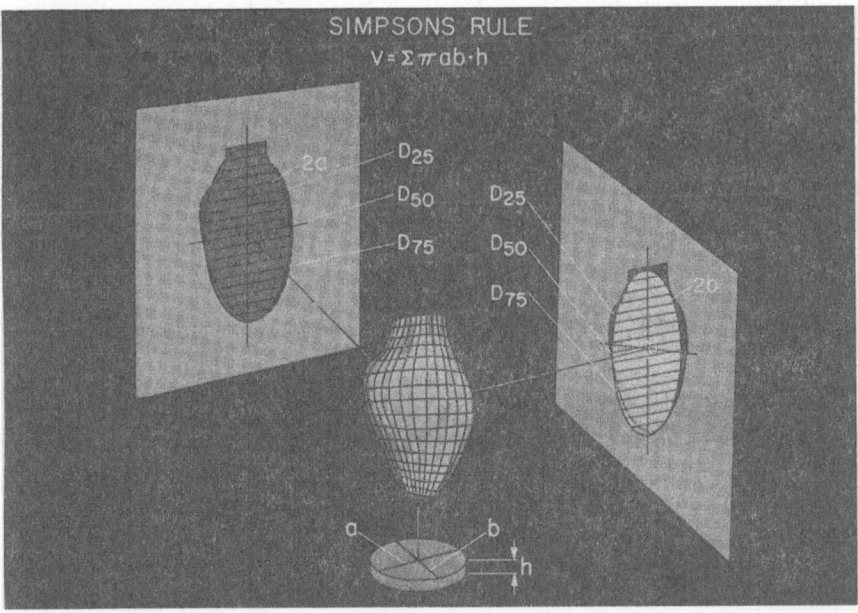

Fig. 4. Method for determining size and shape changes from angiocardiographic films (Simpson's Rule method). 2a, 2b represent respective ventricular diameters for films. D_{25}, D_{50}, D_{75} represent 25th, 50th, 75 th respective diameters for 100 slices of chamber. h represents thickness of a given slice.

cerning ventricular shape. In this latter case the ventricle is usually divided into 100 slices using the apex to aortic valve length of the chamber. The 25th, 50th and 75th diameters are then plotted with respect to time in the cardiac cycle. Such plots are used to describe normal changes in ventricular shape and those caused by non-contracting or akinetic segments. The sum of all slices can be used to calculate LVV as shown. The tedium required to manually analyze changes for 100 of such slices or even four slices is obvious and the magnitude of such procedures becomes more obvious when it is realized that 50 to 150 of such images are required to describe shape changes for a typical cine angiocardiographic study. It became clear when these methods were applied in the study of large numbers of patients that they could be utilized only if assisted by some automatic system such as a computer.

Methods for easily entering radiographic images into the computer for subsequent analysis have not yet been developed. Manual measurements are always possible and serve as a periodic check on computer based methods but are extremely limited due to the time required and possible errors, particularly when large numbers of frames or numbers of patients are involved. Various techniques have been tried to remedy this situation and have consisted of electronic planimeters, manual digitizers, light pens or automatic scanning devices such as a flying spot scanner (15). These methods still require considerable amounts of interaction on the part of the investigator. Recently, video techniques have been used and show great promise. Figure 5 shows the process presently used in this laboratory. The margins of the opacified image are manually traced by means of a digitizer using 8″ ×

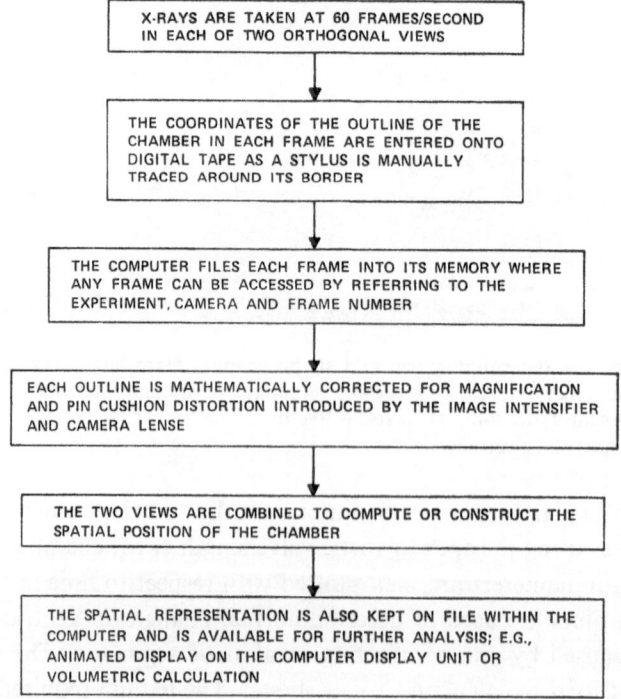

Fig. 5. Method for determining ventricular volumes by computer assisted techniques.

10″ prints made from 35 mm or 16 mm films or directly from the projected images of such films as shown in figure 6. The digitizer produces a digital magnetic tape which is read into an IBM 360/50-computer where they are stored on file for subsequent analysis. The digitized outlines of the chamber

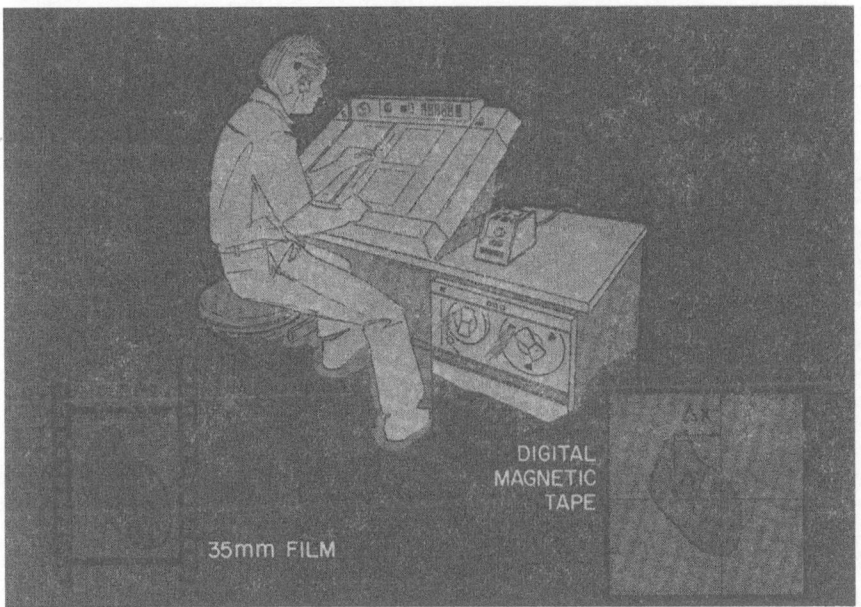

Fig. 6. Calma 303 Digitizer used to manually enter heart outlines into the computer.

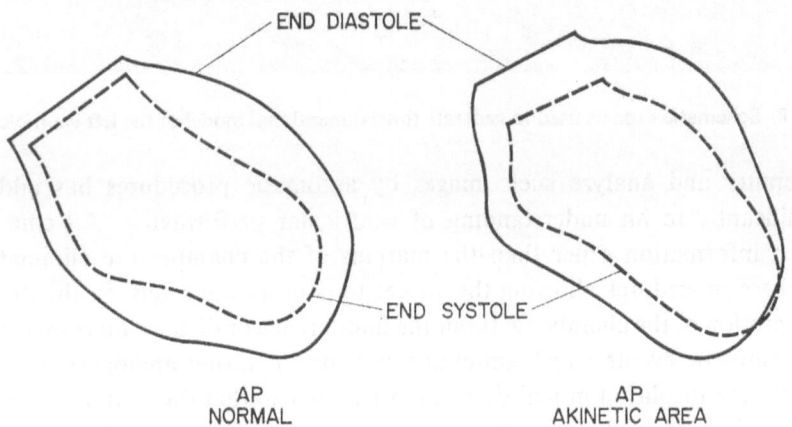

Fig. 7. Heart outlines in the antero-posterior (*A-P*) projection for a normal subject and subject with akinetic area.

can then be viewed in real time on a television screen or analyzed for size and shape changes as outlined above. Figure 7 illustrates typical heart outlines obtained by these procedures for a normal subject and a subject with an akinetic area in the antero-lateral LV wall. If simultaneously recorded, orthogonal images are also recorded, or if images are recorded at some known other projection for the ventricle, three dimensional representations can also be obtained (24); this process is schematically illustrated in figure 8; the results are shown in figure 9. The ability to enter LV outlines into the

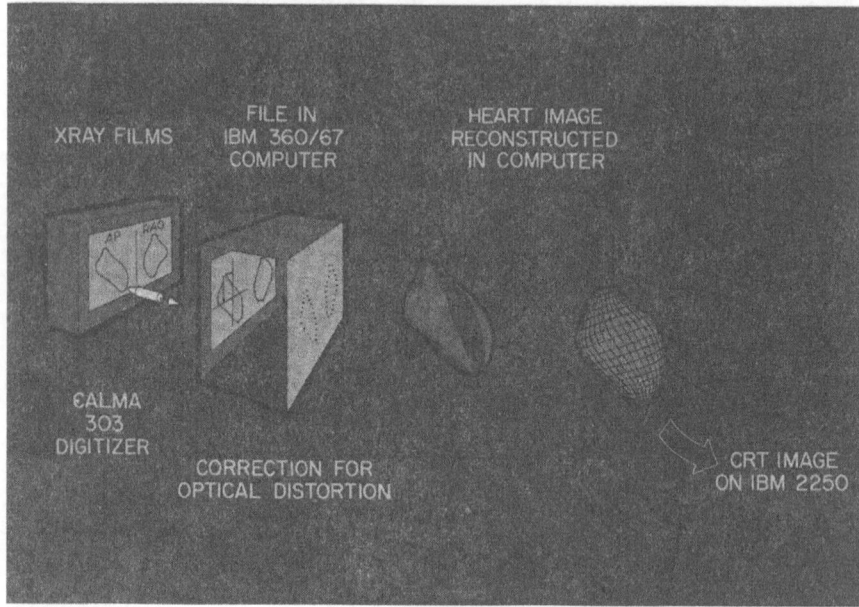

Fig. 8. Schematic process used to generate three dimensional model of the left ventricle.

computer and analyze such images by automatic procedures has added significantly to an understanding of ventricular performance. All cine or video information other than the margins of the chamber are eliminated by these procedures allowing the viewer to concentrate solely on the dynamic motion of the chamber without the interference or distraction from other structures or events which simultaneously occur during angiography. The images are displayed in real time and are stored so that they can be slowed, hastened or stopped as needed. The images can be rotated on the television screen so as to be viewed from different perspectives; this is particularly advantageous with three dimensional representations of the chamber. Isolated sections can be magnified or viewed apart from the rest of the image for intense study. Lastly, images can be displayed with simultaneously recorded hydraulic or mechanical information for dynamic correlations.

Such studies are being used to evaluate subjects for coronary or valvular corrective surgery and subsequent to surgery to analyze their post-operative course. These procedures have been most valuable in studying subjects with coronary artery disease where they are being used to evaluate sections of the ventricular wall which may be akinetic or aneurysmal.

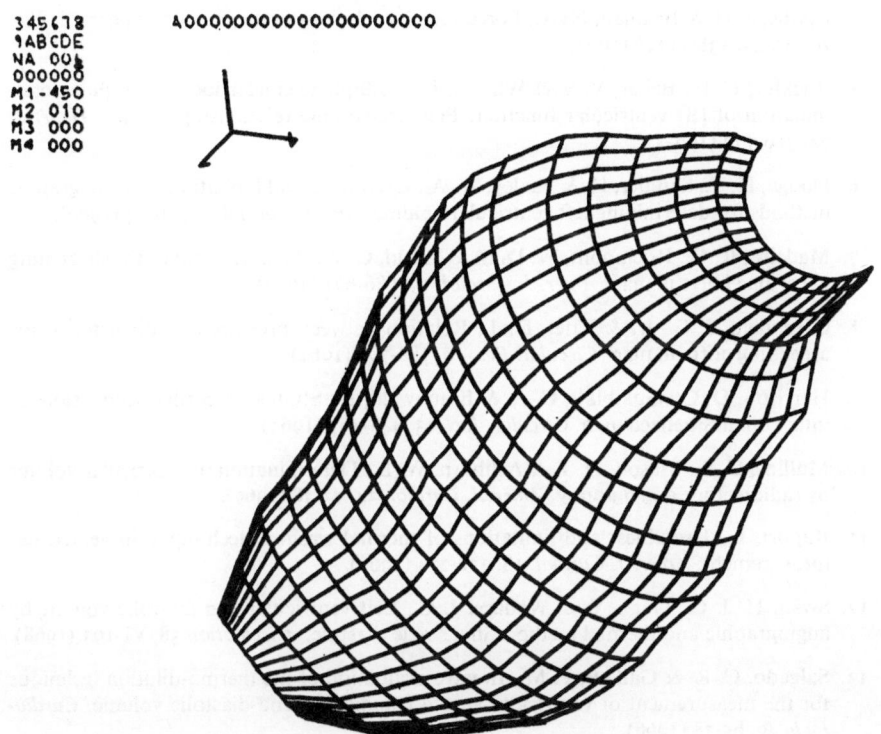

Fig. 9. Computer generated three dimensional model of the left ventricle.

In conclusion it may now be clearly stated that the use of radiographic methods has allowed for quantitation of the hydraulic and mechanical performance of the heart. Advances in computer technology has markedly assisted in analyzing the results of such radiographic procedures and holds promise for making such data available in real time on-line at the time of routine heart catheterization procedures.

REFERENCES

1. Covell, J. W., Ross, J. jr. & Sonnenblick, E. H., Comparison of the force velocity relation and ventricular function curves as a measure of the contractile state of the intact heart. *Circulat. Res.* 19, 364-372 (1966).

2. Fry, D. L., Griggs, D. M. & Greenfield, J. C., Myocardial mechanics: Tension-celocity-length relationships of heart muscle. *Circulat. Res.* 14, 73-85 (1964).

3. Gault, J. H., Ross, J. jr. & Braunwald, E., Contractile state of the left ventricle in man, instantaneous tension-velocity-length relationships in patients with and without disease of the left ventricular myocardium. *Circulat. Res.* 22, 451-463 (1968).

4. Levine, J. H. & Britman, N. A., Force velocity relations in the intact dog heart. *J. clin. Invest.* 43, 1383-1396 (1964).

5. Rackley, C. E., Behar, V. S. & Whalen, R. E., Biplane cineangiocardiographic determination of left ventricular function: Pressure-volume relationships. *Amer. Heart J.* 74, 766-779 (1967).

6. Dodge, H. T., Sandler, H. & Baxley, W. A., Usefulness and limitations of radiographic methods for determining left ventricular volume. *Am. J. Cardiol.* 18, 10-24 (1966).

7. Madeira, R. G., Rochmont, W. D. M. & Gadd, C. W., Measurement of the shortening of cardiac fibers in man. *Amer. J. Cardiol.* 19, 686-691 (1967).

8. Greenfield, J. C., jr. & Patel, D. J., Relation between pressure and diameter in the ascending aorta in man. *Circulat. Res.* 10, 788-781 (1962).

9. Harrison, D. C., Goldblatt, C. A. & Braunwald, E., Studies on cardiac dimensions in intact unanesthetized man. *Circulat. Res.* 13, 448-467 (1963).

10. Mullins, C. B., Mason, D. T. & Ashburn, W. L., Determination of ventricular volume by radioisotope angiography. *Amer. J. Cardiol.* 24, 72-78 (1969).

11. Raport, E., Usefulness and limitations of thermal washout techniques in ventricular measurement. *Amer. J. Cardiol.* 18, 226-234 (1966).

12. Swan, H. J. C., Ganz, V. & Wallace, J. C., Left ventricular end-diastolic volume by angiographic and thermal methods in a single diastole. *Circulation* 38, VI-193 (1968).

13. Salgado, C. R. & Galletti, P. M., In vitro evaluation of the thermo-dilution technique for the measurement of ventricular stroke volume and end-diastolic volume. *Cardiologia* 49, 65-78 (1966).

14. Hugenholtz, P. G., Wagner, H. R. & Sandler, H., The in vivo determination of left ventricular volume. Comparison of the fiber optic indicator dilution and the angiocardiographic methods. *Circulation* 37, 489-508 (1969).

15. Sandler, H., Dimensional analysis of the heart – a review. *Amer. J. med. Sci.* 260, 56-65 (1970).

16. Dodge, H. T., Sandler, H. & Ballew, D. W., The use of biplane angiocardiography for measurement of left ventricular volume in man. *Amer. Heart J.* 60, 762-776 (1960).

17. Rackley, C. E., Dodge, H. T. & Coble, Y. D., A method for determining left ventricular mass in man. *Circulation* 29, 666 (1964).

18. Dodge, H. T., Hay, R. E. & Sandler, H., Pressure-volume of the diastolic left ventricle of man with heart disease. *Amer. Heart J.* 64, 503-11 (1962).

19. Baxley, W. A. & Dodge, H. T., Relationship of left ventricle performance and hypertrophy in humans. In: Alpert, N. R. (ed.), *Cardiac Hypertrophy.* pp. 425-431. New York (N.Y.) 1971.

20. McDonald, I. G., Shape and movements of the human left ventricle during systole. *Amer. J. Cardiol.* 26, 221-230 (1970).

21. Popp, R. L. & Harrison, D. C., Ultrasonic cardiac echography for determining stroke volume and valvular regurgitation. *Circulation* 41, 493-502 (1970).

22. Kennedy, J. W., Reickenbach, D. D. & Baxley, W. A., Left ventricular mass. *Amer. J. Cardiol.* 19, 221-223 (1967).

23. Rackley, C. W., Dear, H. D. & Baxley, W. A., Left ventricular dilatation and hypertrophy in coronary artery disease. In: Alpert, N.R. (ed.), Cardiac hypertrophy. pp. 453-465. New York (N.Y.) 1971.

24. Sandler, H. & Rasmussen, D., Angiographic analysis of heart geometry. In: Heintzen, P. N. (ed.), *Roentgen-, cine- and videodensitometry.* pp. 212-224. Stuttgart 1971.

MEASUREMENT OF
CONTRACTILE ELEMENT VELOCITY
A COMPARISON OF THREE METHODS

G. T. MEESTER, J. ROELANDT AND P. G. HUGENHOLTZ

According to Maxwell's model, a myocardial muscle fiber is represented by a combination of three mechanical components. The contractile element is arranged in series with one elastic element, while the second elastic element is coupled in parallel to the other two.

With incremental loading of a myocardial muscle strip, the contracting velocity declines exponentially. Curves of force versus velocity show that peak velocity is reached at an early phase of contraction. The force-velocity curve can be extrapolated to a point of zero force where velocity reaches a hypothetical maximal value (V_{max}). This value V_{max} is thought to reflect the contractile state of a given muscle strip, and is independent of the after-load and preload imposed on cardiac muscle during contraction.

Studies on isolated cat papillary muscle have demonstrated that this relationship between V_{max} and the contractile state exist for cardiac muscle (Sonnenblick c.s.).

Measurement of contractile element velocity (V_{CE}) in the intact heart is also possible, again based on the three-element model.

In this study, three methods for obtaining V_{max} have been applied in the experimental animal (pigs) and results are compared for a great variety of loading conditions.

V_{CE} CALCULATED FROM PRESSURE

The left ventricular pressure signal alone can be used as a means of calculating V_{CE}. During the isometric phase of systole the size and shape of the left ventricle may be assumed to be constant, provided there is no dyskinetic movement. According to the three-component model, V_{CE} equals in this phase the velocity of elongation of the series elastic element (V_{SE}). This elastic element, has exponential stress-length characteristics expressed as:

$V_{SE} = (dT/dt)/K.T$ where $T = $ stress

$K = $ elasticity modulus

In isometric contraction stress is equal to pressure (P) times a geometric constant (C).

$V_{SE} = C. (dP/dt)/K.C.P.$

$V_{CE} = (dP/dt)/K.P.$

The value K is comprised of geometric and elastic properties and is probably between 28 and 40. For direct comparison in the same animal it can be assumed to be constant and is set $K = 1$ in this study.

Developed force also bears a direct relationship to intracavity pressure when no geometrical changes are present. In this way the force-velocity curve during isovolumetric systole can be derived from the pressure signal alone. Left ventricular pressure should be measured with a catheter-tip manometer to exclude phase or frequency response distortion.

Force-velocity curves can be calculated from the pressure signal completely by hand, with a small analogue device or with a digital computer.

Manual processing is time-consuming and tedious. With the analogue device, consisting of a logarithmic amplifier and differentiator, the dP/dt/P expression can be calculated and displayed versus the pressure signal as a loop on a X-Y oscilloscope. The loop is then photographed. With a digital computer the process can be automated completely. V_{max} is extrapolated in a more objective way by least squares fit of a straight line descending slope between fixed limits of pressure within isovolumic systole. Representative values are printed out.

V_{CE} CAN ALSO BE MEASURED FROM THE MOVEMENTS OF THE VENTRIC-ULAR WALL ITSELF

In our study silver clips were implanted in the left ventricular wall of experimental animals in such a way that a line joining them was parallel to the RAO plane, minimizing the errors resulting from rotation of the heart during the cardiac cycle. In this way several markers were implanted: one at the apex, one between the aortic and mitral valves and one at the anterior and posterior free surfaces of the left ventricle.

Clip movement is measured in successive frames of the cine-radiogram (80 fr/sec). Instantaneous length between markers is plotted versus synchronous intraventricular pressure both for control measurements and for interventions.

THE LEFT VENTRICULAR (CINE) ANGIOGRAM PROVIDES A THIRD
MEANS OF DETERMINING V_{CE}

Left ventricular volume calculated from the contours of LV images, via the area-length method, combined with instantaneous LV pressure and wall thickness permits calculation of several parameters (midwall stress, stroke volume, ejection fraction). V_{CE} based on midwall stress can then be derived and shown graphically.

These three methods have their own specific advantages and limitations. The injected contrast medium in the angio-stress method acts as an extra volume load and may exert a negative inotropic influence.

The contrast medium has been shown to influence contractility when the coronary circulation is perfused, starting 5-6 beats after injection in the left ventricle. To exclude this effect calculations were limited to the first three consecutive beats after injection.

Pressure-derived V_{CE} is by definition limited to isovolumetric ventricular systole. The pressure of mitral regurgitation does not influence this parameter as regurgitant flow will reach significant levels only in later phases of systole while peak V_{CE} is reached in the first 30-40 milliseconds.

Markers enable follow-up of V_{CE} determinations over longer periods without any disturbing influences. They are however at present confined to the experimental laboratory since their introduction necessitates thoracotomy.

In this study V_{CE} and other parameters were measured under a wide variety of conditions. All three methods were applied in the same beat. The interventions consist of changes in preload, afterload and contractility. This was effectuated by balloon insufflation in the inferior vena cava, rapid infusion of 2 ml/kg bodyweight saline and administration of angiotensin and isoprenalin. After each of these interventions measurements were carried out and comparisons made with the control state. Results show good agreement between V_{max} determinations from the three methods discussed, as shown in the table below.

The angio- and pressure-derived data are extremely compatible, while clip data show greater spread. This may result from the limited number of clips providing only three measured lengths per image.

It can be concluded that these silver markers have no impeding effect on left ventricular contraction, as indicated by V_{max}. All data given in table I are expressed in units of sec^{-1} since K has been dropped.

Table 1.

V_{max} (sec^{-1}) (Pressure derived)	V_{max} (sec^{-1}) (Angio-stress)	V_{max} (sec^{-1}) (Clip movement)
59	63	
53	54	
57	58	
49	50	
39	40	
65	62	
49	48	49
64	62	64
52	52	52
62	61	62
62	63	64
55	55	57
45	44	47
58	46	55
53	54	49
59	58	58
111		109

CONCLUSIONS

1. Normal values for V_{max} in the anaesthesized pig are 53-64 second^{-1}. (K = 1).
2. The investigated methods of V_{CE} determination based on stress, intracavitary pressure and marker movement show good agreement.
3. Implanted silver markers do not exert a negative effect on left ventricular contraction as measured by V_{max}.
4. Long-term measurements of V_{CE} can be effectuated by recording silver clip movements.

DETERMINATION OF LEFT VENTRICULAR VOLUME AND EJECTION FRACTION BY ECHOCARDIOGRAPHY*

E. CRAIGE, N. J. FORTUIN, M. E. SHERMAN AND W. P. HOOD JR.

In the past few years remarkable advances have been made in accuracy of cardiac diagnosis by external graphic techniques. The latest of these, echocardiography, differs from previous methods in that it penetrates the surface of the chest to provide information regarding movements of ventricular walls, septum and valves. It offers the opportunity to obtain quantitative data on cardiac function without trauma or risk to the patient.

The basic principle underlying the use of echocardiographic techniques is that an ultrasonic beam directed through the body will be reflected backward or echoed when tissues of differing acoustic impedance are met, for instance heart muscle and blood. Because the speed of sound in tissue is known, the elapsed time between transmission and subsequent reception of a signal allows calculations of the distance between the ultrasonic source and the tissue interface.

In figure 1, the technique for obtaining minor axis dimensions by echocardiography is demonstrated utilizing a diagrammatic representation of a horizontal section through the thorax. The heart chambers are labelled. The ultrasonic transducer is placed in the fourth or fifth intercostal space just to the left of the sternum. This transducer both transmits the ultrasonic beam and receives the resultant echoes. The characteristic motion of the anterior leaflet of the mitral valve is detected by directing the sonic beam posteriorly and slightly medially as shown. The beam is then directed slightly laterally and inferiorly away from the mitral valve until a plane is found in which movements of the interventricular septum and posterior left ventricular wall which are highly characteristic, are noted.

A study of the geometry of left ventricular contraction using angiographic techniques in the normal and pathologic human heart, recently completed in

* Supported by the U.S. Environmental Protection Agency, Research Triangle Park, North Carolina and the Henry A. Foscue Professorship at the University of North Carolina in Chapel Hill, N.C.

our laboratory has demonstrated that 80-90% of left ventricular stroke volume can be accounted for by changes in the minor axis of the chamber during systole (1). The long, or apex to base, axis changes relatively little during the cardiac cycle and therefore plays a smaller role in left ventricular

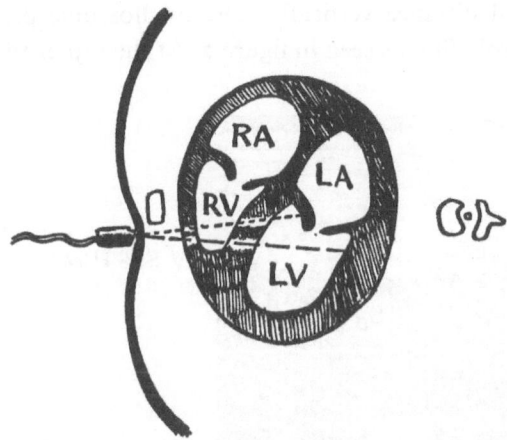

Fig. 1. Cross section through the heart at the level of the mitral valve to show paths traversed by echo beams. Sternum and echo transducer are to the left, spine to the right. Short dashed line represents path of echo beam to the anterior mitral valve leaflet. Lateral and inferior movement of transducer results in an ultrasonic path which passes through chest wall, right ventricular wall, interventricular septum, and posterior left ventricular wall successively, as indicated by line with longer dashes. Figures 1-4 are reprinted from *Circulation* with permission of the authors (2), editor, and the American Heart Association, Inc.

ejection. A number of investigators have previously made similar observations in the canine heart. Because of this, it seemed likely that measurement of the minor ventricular axis by a non-invasive method might provide important correlative information about left ventricular volumes and ejection fraction (2). Such a non-invasive method has become available through the use of ultrasonic echocardiography (3, 4, 5).

We performed the present investigations to validate the use of echo-measured dimensions as correlates of left ventricular volume. These studies were designed to answer the following specific question: 1. What is the relationship between minor axis dimensions measured by echocardiography in systole and diastole and those obtained from angiocardiograms? 2. What is the relationship between the echo-measured dimensions and left ventricular volumes? and 3. Can ventricular volumes be derived from the echo dimensions alone?

To answer these questions we obtained echocardiograms for measurement
of minor axis ventricular dimensions in 26 patients who also had left ventricular volumes measured by angiocardiography.

Motion of the interventricular system and posterior left ventricular wall is
displayed on an oscilloscope in a manner in which time is represented
horizontally and distance vertically. The oscilloscopic picture is then recorded on polaroid film as seen in figure 2. At the top of the graphic record

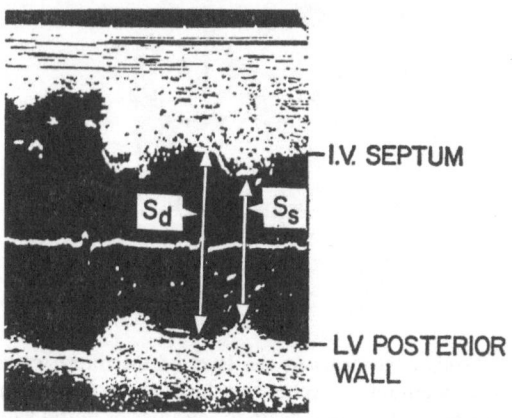

Fig. 2. Technique for measuring minor axis dimensions from echocardiogram. Echocardiogram was obtained by directing ultrasonic beam as described in figure 1. Cf. text for details.

the ultrasonic signal from the chest wall is seen, at the bottom the signal from
the posterior left ventricular wall. The septum lies in between these echoes
and can be seen to move posteriorly away from the chest wall during ventricular systole while the posterior wall moves toward the chest wall. End-
diastolic minor axis dimensions are measured at the peak of the R wave of
the simultaneously displayed electrocardiogram as indicated by the arrow
labelled S_D and end-systolic dimensions at the point where the septum and
posterior ventricular wall approach each other as indicated by S_S. The per
cent minor axis change with systole or echo ejection fraction is determined by
subtracting end-systolic from end-diastolic dimension and dividing by the
end-diastolic dimension.

Cardiac catheterization and biplane angiocardiography with films recorded
at 6 or 8 per second for measurement of the left ventricular volumes were
performed within 24 hours of obtaining the echo measurements in the 23
patients studied. Left ventricular volumes were computed by the length-area
method of Dodge and associates (6). Minor axis dimensions were derived

rather than measured from the planimetered area of the left ventricle assuming an ellipsoidal reference figure (7). The mean of minor axis dimensions obtained in this manner from each pair of AP and lateral films was taken as the minor axis of an idealized prolate ellipsoid.

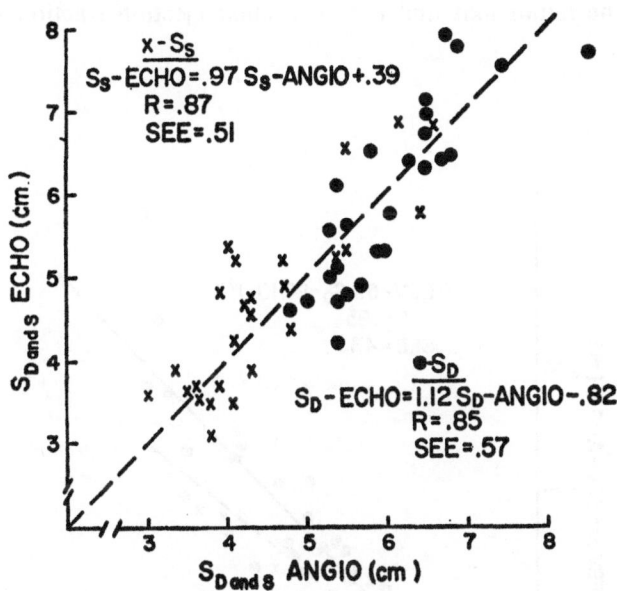

Fig. 3. Comparison of minor axis dimensions in systole (S$_S$-X's) and diastole (S$_D$-solid dots) determined by echocardiography and angiocardiography. Dashed line is line of identity. R = correlation coefficient, SEE = standard error of the estimate.

In figure 3, the relationship between echo measured end-systolic and end-diastolic minor axes, represented on the vertical axis, is compared with minor axes derived from angiocardiograms, on the horizontal axis. The systolic dimensions are represented by X's, the diastolic dimensions by solid dots; the dashed line is the line of identity. In both cases there is a highly significant relationship between dimensions obtained by the two techniques, the correlation coefficient being slightly better for systolic dimensions. There is a tendency for a slight overestimation of end-systolic dimensions with the echo technique and a slight underestimation of end-diastolic dimensions. This results in an underestimate of the per cent change in the minor axis with systole.

In figure 4, echo dimensions represented on the horizontal axis are compared with end-systolic and end-diastolic volumes determined by angiocardiography and shown on the vertical axis. The solid line and dots represent end-diastolic measurements, the broken line and X's those at end-systole. The correlation coefficients between dimensions and volumes are highly significant and slightly better at end-systole than end-diastole. There is also a significant correlation between the echo ejection fraction or per cent change in the minor axis and left ventricular ejection fraction with an R value of .79.

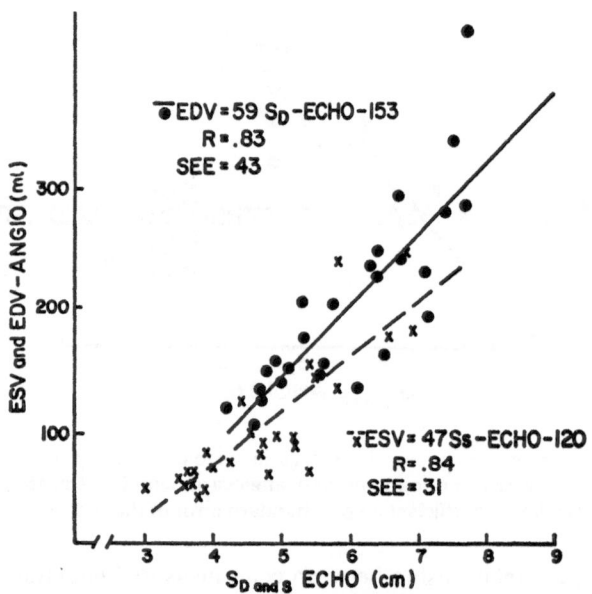

Fig. 4. Comparison of echo measured minor axis dimensions with angiographic end-systolic (ESV-x's) and end-diastolic (EDV-solid dots) volumes. Solid and dashed lines are least squares regression lines for variables.

We derived formulae for prediction of end-systolic and end-diastolic volumes from echo dimensions alone utilizing the regression date shown in figure 4. The formula for derivation of end-diastolic volume is shown in the upper left of this figure, that for end-systolic volume in the lower right.

Left ventricular volumes were then derived from the echo data by means of these equations and compared with volumes determined by angiocardio-

graphy as shown in figure 5. Again end-systolic volumes are represented by
X's and end-diastolic volumes by solid dots; the dashed line is the line of
identity. Volumes derived from the echo dimensions by regression formulae
are represented on the vertical axis and those determined from the angio

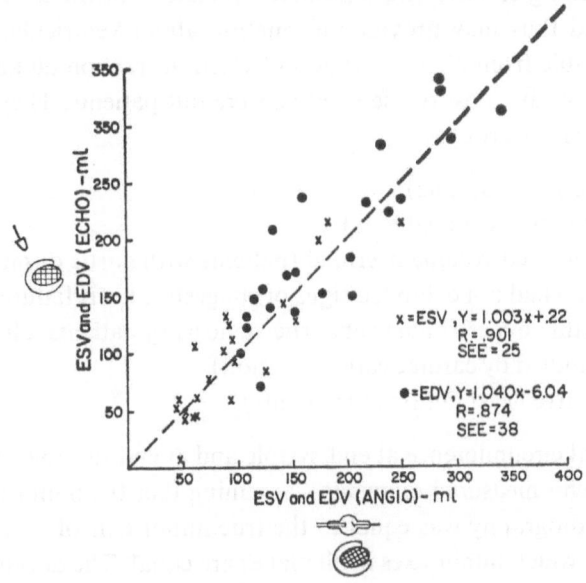

Fig. 5. Comparison of angiographic ventricular volumes with those derived from echo
dimensions.

cardiograms on the horizontal axis. There is an excellent correlation between
the derived and measured volumes over a wide range of end-systolic and
end-diastolic volumes. This is reflected in the high R values and the approximation of the regression equations to the line of identity. Left ventricular
stroke volume, which is determined by subtracting end-systolic from end-
diastolic volume also shows a good correlation between derived and measured values with an R value of .77. From this part of our studies, then we
have attempted to validate the use of left ventricular dimensions determined
by echocardiography as correlates of left ventricular volumes by comparing
echo-measured dimensions with volumes determined by angiocardiography.
We have shown that the echo-measured minor axis dimensions resemble true
minor axis dimensions, that there are highly significant correlations between
echo dimensions and ventricular volumes, and that from this relationship

equations can be derived which allow accurate prediction of ventricular volumes and ejection fraction from the echo data alone.

In addition to this use of echo measured dimensions, I would like to describe in this report another parameter of ventricular function which can be determined by the echo technique, the mean velocity of circumferential fiber shortening or VCF. This parameter is related to cardiac muscle function directly and thus may provide information about ventricular performance not obtainable from a consideration of ejection fraction alone (8). For this part of the study, most of the subjects were out patients. They were divided into five separate groups:

I. Normals (10 subjects)
II. Mitral stenosis (13 patients)
III. Compensated volume overload (patients with aortic or mitral regurgitation who had not exhibited signs of congestive heart failure)
IV. Idiopathic hypertrophic subaortic stenosis (5 patients, all of whom had been studied by cardiac catheterization)
V. Congestive heart failure (17 patients)

The internal circumference at end-systole and at end-diastole are determined from the echo-measured diameter – assuming that the minor axis measured by echocardiography was equal to the true minor axis of an ellipsoid of revolution in which minor axes in all planes are equal. The duration of circumferential shortening is measured from the onset of anterior movement of the posterior wall to its peak.

In figure 6, the mean velocity of circumferential fiber shortening in the several groups of patients is compared. Shortening is expressed not in centimeters but in circumferences per second which permits a better comparison between the large volume hearts seen in Group III – compensated volume overload – and normals. The patients in Group III – with aortic and mitral regurgitation, compensated, have a VCF which is not significantly different from normals.

Group II (mitral stenosis) was only slightly decreased from normal and Group V (congestive heart failure) markedly diminished.

An excessive velocity of circumferential fiber shortening was seen in the patients with idiopathic hypertrophic subaortic stenosis.

Two patients in Group V overlapped with normal group. Both had valvular heart disease and in one the valvular lesion was relatively acute (aortic regurgitation secondary to infective endocarditis without known previous heart disease). While both of these subjects had circulatory congestion as a result of overwhelming volume loads to the left ventricle, it is possible that their cardiac muscle function may have been quite adequate. Several patients in Group III fell below the range of normals and thus, though asymptomatic, may have abnormal left ventricular function.

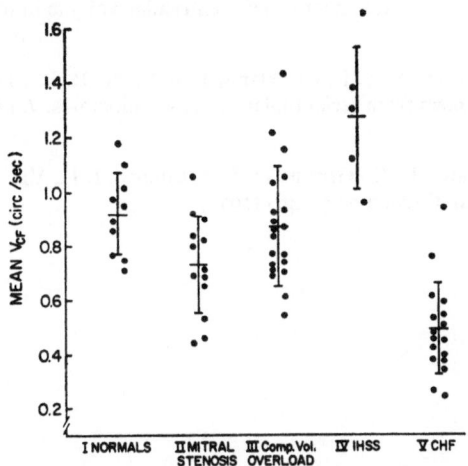

Fig. 6. Values for mean circumferential shortening velocity (VCF) in patient groups.

This type of information about left ventricular function has before now been obtained only by invasive methods. The echo study however can be accomplished painlessly at low cost, repeatedly and without danger to the patient. The information obtained is closely related to that obtained from angiographic studies. Further studies comparing the method with invasively determined measurements will be necessary precisely to determine the sensitivity of the method. It is likely that this method will prove more sensitive than other existing non-invasive techniques for the evaluation of left ventricular function.

REFERENCES

1. Hood, W. P. jr. & Rolett, E., Patterns of contraction in the human left ventricle. *Circulation* 40 (Suppl III), 109 (1969).

2. Fortuin, N. J., Hood, W. P. jr., Sherman, M. E. & Craige, E., Determination of left ventricular volumes by ultrasound. *Circulation* 44, 575 (1971).

3. Popp, R. L., Wolfe, S. B., Hirata, T. & Feigenbaum, H., Estimation of right and left ventricular size by ultrasound. *Amer. J. Cardiol.* 24, 523 (1969).

4. Popp, R. L. & Harrison, D. C., Ultrasonic cardiac echography for determining stroke volume and valvular regurgitation. *Circulation* 41, 493 (1970).

5. Chapelle, M. & Mensch, B., Etude des variations du diamètre ventriculaire gauche chez l'homme par echocardiographie transthoracique. *Arch. Mal. Coeur* 62, 1505 (1969).

6. Dodge, H. T., Sandler, H., Ballew, D. W. & Lord, J. D. jr, The use of biplane angio-cardiography for the measurement of left ventricular volume in man. *Amer. Heart. J.* 60, 762 (1960).

7. Rackley, C. E., Hood, W. P. jr, Cleveland, L. & Stacy, R. W., Derivation of cardiac mechanical parameters from serial biplane angiocardiograms. *J. appl. Physiol.* 24, 254 (1968).

8. Falsetti, H. L., Mates, R. E., Greene, D. B. & Bunnell, I. L., V_{Max} as an index of con-tractile state in man. *Circulation* 43, 467 (1971).

DISCUSSION

Schaper: I have a question for Dr. Sandler: you showed very beautifully that the diastolic pressure-volume relationship is not necessarily constant as we find stated in textbooks of physiology and cardiology. I am prepared to call this a variable diastolic tone. Do you think that this is the correct word for this condition and secondly is it a functional state or rather a structural alteration or a diseased state? How does this concept of a variable diastolic tone fit into the framework of the dimensions which determine contractility? Is it a kind of fifth dimension? Furthermore, has it perhaps something to do with coronary perfusion? I have recently observed that an increased coronary flow as well as decreased coronary flow can change the compliance of the ventricular wall. That means that the heart looks very much like a kind of erectile tissue.

Sandler: Lets look at the heart as a pump *and* as a muscle. Dr. Brutsaert put down some of the things which we are talking about, force, length, velocity and time. What we like to do as physicians is to make things very simple. No clinician at a patient's bedside wants to accept the fact that we cannot give him *one* number that characterized the patient's status. It is almost like taking a trip looking for the Holy Grail. You don't want to think of this as a complex system. You want one number and that everything else will be solved from this time on. Unfortunately it is *not* that way. It turns out that this is a five dimensional system. Each item on the pump side has an equivalent or analogous situation in terms of muscle function. We have the wall stress which Dr. Hugenholtz talked about, which is equivalent to force. We have volume which is equivalent to length, we have flow which is related to impedance and equivalent to pre-load and after-load and we have time or the electrocardiogram which is related to time of activation and we have efficiency of energy utilization which is related to oxygen consumption which is identical in both systems. There is no known parameter or set of parameters at this time which states or relates that everything is in equilibrium. There is nothing to make me think that the heart becomes disequilibrated between the muscle and the fluid at any time. If you have five variables, as we have here, most researchers have given up hope of arriving at a reasonable answer by seeking interrelationships between them all but have sought answers by looking at changes in a single parameter. Dr. Brutsaert elegantly demonstrated how this latter system can produce important information. He presented data on phase-plane plots of muscle length. Such plots embody the concepts of looking at a variable with respect to the rate of change of that same variable. He also showed a diagram in which velocity of length change and length were compared, but velocity is really the rate of change of length and such a comparison results in a loop termed a phase-plane plot. Change in contractile state is known to clearly alter the rate of force and length changes from the resting state. Taking a derivative amplifies these changes. This approach has been most widely used with the recorded pressure pulse. Here dP/dt has been compared to various points on the phase-plane plot or extrapolation from these plots have been used to identify the contractile state of the myocardium.

With this background, I would now like to return to your question about what happens during the diastolic pressure volume loop. You want to look at the graph of pressure versus volume at a specific time or over a specific time during diastole. Compliance would be the slope of this curve or the change in pressure with respect to volume. What we demonstrated earlier in this meeting is that with chronic heart disease the pressure volume characteristics of the left ventricle changes. During acute experiments, we do not see this. Particularly in the laboratory, there seems to be a reasonably linear relationship between pressure and volume. When chronic disease occurs, however, this changes. When in the disease course this begins and how the disease process works to produce it is not known. I do know that in biopsy specimens from various people we find various kinds of diffuse fibrotic processes which are not present in the normal heart. Undoubtedly the presence of fibrosis in the wall of the heart will change its pressure-volume characteristics. Whether this occurs solely on the basis of coronary artery perfusion is unknown to me. I would guess that it would respond to such changes. What I do know is that we require 5 dimensions in order to characterize heart performance. Anyone who uses one dimension or two to characterize the five is in for trouble. What I mean by this is that we may do an experiment and not find pressure-volume change; this does not mean function is unchanged. What I think we can do is to make the computer do a lot of rational simplifications for us. This is one of the aspects where we should not get lazy. I think we shall have a system which can do this in the near future. When all primary parameters are measured, measured correctly and acceptable, we shall have the answers or solutions to these puzzling problems.

Audience: We see a large number of people with kinetic segments and with what looks like a satisfactorily functioning ventricle and yet with a fairly elevated end-diastolic pressure. Do you think that this has anything to do with the diastolic compliance or is this just a failure of the ventricle? Can we establish a direct relationship between the pressure and cardiac failure in some sense or with the mean left atrial pressure or with whatever pressure you want?

Meester: It is rather difficult to answer your question. Dr. Hugenholtz suggested the pacing situation. When you pace a patient in the atrial pacing stress test and increase heart rate, I would not expect the diastolic compliance to change. However, diastolic pressure does go up, especially in the case of coronary heart disease. We have not many data on volume at the same time but we have evidence that compliance changes under these circumstances. I personally do not feel that diastolic tone plays a large role but I can't state what role it does play.

Hugenholtz: We observed the end-diastolic pressure to go up until the point of pain, when we stopped the test. We have the feeling that these hearts do not change their performance appropriately. It does indeed look as if at times there is a massive compliance change, the same kind that has been noted experimentally by Schaper.

Brutsaert: I think that the question raised is of the utmost importance at this time. I agree with Dr. Sandler that all of the parameters, that we have been measuring during the contraction, continue during relaxation and diastole in the resting muscle. In skeletal muscle it has been shown recently that there is a clear-cut diastolic tonus. Why should there then be no diastolic tonus or resting activity in heart muscle? The group of Beneken and Donders of the Institute of Medical Physics have been using an analogue model in which they assumed diastolic tonus to be active. Their simulated computer data fit very well with our experimental data.

Hugenholtz: Mr. Donders could you comment on that, particularly in relation to the work that was done by Monroe and others who have stated that there is an active cost (in terms of oxygen) in relaxation after contraction?

Donders: Most of the models of cardiac muscle mechanics, which exist at this moment, fail at the transition point between the resting state and the activated state. Usually, it is assumed that the contractile element (CE) at rest is freely extensible and exerts no force, which means that the analogue model has only elastic properties at rest. This is in contradiction with the visco-elastic behaviour of almost all biological tissues, including the resting heart muscle.

G. Pollack analysed E. H. Sonnenblick's data in terms of a three element model, but neglected the contribution of the CE at rest. He concluded that V_{max} is a function of initial muscle length, in contradiction to Sonnenblick's own conclusions. However, assuming a contractile element which exerts a certain resting force, the preload upon the CE is unequal to zero at the start of the contraction and therefore Pollack's analysis is no longer valid.

The assumption of the viscous nature of the CE at rest implies that the filling rate of the ventricle is limited intrinsically, which makes the diastolic viscous properties of the ventricle an important parameter of muscle contraction.

The decay of the active state is most probably a continuous multi-exponential decay which continues during diastole until a new contraction starts. There may always be a residual interaction between the actin and myosin filaments, as is demonstrated for the skeletal muscle at rest by D. K. Hill.

The consequence of a resting force exerted by the CE is that the discrepancy between the 'Voigt' and 'Maxwell' type of three element models is less significant and both tend toward a simple two element model since the contribution of the parallel elastic element is negligible in the normal working range.

Heintzen: It may be that this resting activity has a certain constant value and that it is not influenced by the disease or by certain drugs. This could mean that it could be a parameter for the whole evaluation or it could be a constant. Another parameter brought up by Dr. Schaper which should perhaps be re-introduced into this discussion is the ventricular resting compliance.

Audience: I would like each member of the panel to define contractility in his own words and to state which parameters in judging cardiac function of contractility or other parameters he would like to have measured.

Hugenholtz: I refuse to answer that question on the grounds that it may 'incriminate' me. There is, however, another reason why I refuse to answer it. I don't think that we should be trapped by such a rhetorical question. This is a fundamental objection on my part. I do not think that this is the way we should approach the problem just as Dr. Sandler pointed out earlier. We do not need one factor to describe contractility but the instantaneous interrelationship of several factors. I would be very happy to give you my present definition of contractility, but not in the sense that it would be the road to 'Heaven'. Therefore, I will say at this point that 'contractility' is a constellation of incompletely defined factors which describe the active state of the muscle. This is just a description and not a definition.

Meester: The term 'contractility' means nothing specific to me at the moment.

Selvester: I think that the term contractility has some use. We have talked about it for years when we did not know what it was. I am not sure that we know what it is now. The work on muscle physiology has at least forced us to look at preload and afterload and then admit that there must be other factors involved besides these. There must be something about the state of the muscle itself that we have to look at and measure. It is not yet known by anyone whether force-velocity relationships are the way to look at it, but that kind of modification seems to be the best thing we have at this time.

Brutsaert: I would define 'contractility' as the relationship between force, velocity and length as a function of time. This applies both to contraction and relaxation and to resting muscle if there is a diastolic tonus. The term 'change in contractility' would then refer to an upward or downward shift of this relationship. This is my point of view as a muscle physiologist. It is purely descriptive and does not consider any analysis of the basic mechanisms involved. An entirely different description would be proposed by a biochemist or an electrophysiologist and would instead be related to excitation-contraction coupling or to what happens to calcium as a function of time, related to the initiation and the maintainance of the contraction of cardiac muscle.

Sandler: It is interesting that contractility is the one aspect of the physiologic state that is not easily describable by engineering or mechanical terms. If one were to look at all of the various ways that an engineer has available to describe the performance of a system, we would not be able to find any one term that would describe the physiological property we call 'contractility'. That is why it is so difficult. Using the systems approach that Dr. Sayers introduced at this conference, we could ask ourselves what are the weighting functions involved? Pressure is by far the most important measurement from this point of view. Several years ago, Monroe showed that 90% of the oxygen consumption of the heart is utilized in raising the pressure from end-diastolic to peak systolic value. Therefore, we know that pressure is of tremendous importance. When there is a change in contractility we also observe a very small increase in peak pressure and change or shortening with respect to time. If we were to take the differential here, dP/dt, it would amplify the small changes that occur. Therefore, if I were looking for something quick, I would use the differential. A comparison of dP/dt and P – a phase plane plot as described previously – should contain a lot of information concerning contractility. From the rest of the factors, I would consider the efficiency of oxygen consumption as the next most important weighted parameter. The comparison of pressure data and oxygen consumption as a measure of contractility should produce a great degree of unique and useful information concerning contractility.

Selvester: I would like to ask Dr. Craige a question which occurred to me during his presentation. The capacity to measure volumes from outside the chest by echocardiography offers interesting possibilities. One of these would be to do serial studies of volumetrics with exercise. Have you had any success in measuring these in exercise either in normals or in coronary patients?

Craige: The only exercise we have used is the isometric handgrip contraction because it is very difficult to get a satisfactory volume record even under the most ideal circumstances.

Audience: It is very common to get different diameters by ultrasound because of the shifting of the angles. What reference points do you use to be certain that you have the same diameters in different patients at different times?

Craige: There are obviously a number of technical problems with this method and I would not wish to minimize them. It is true that you might be changing to a different angle and exaggerate the cross-sectional diameter in a patient. The reference that we use is the mitral valve; then we move the beam slightly laterally and slightly inferior. At that point one picks up the posterior wall. In the same patient at least, it is possible to get reproducible figures. In order to evaluate the validity of the method we have related it to the values obtained in angiography. The relationship appears to be quite good in our experience and others have even higher correlation coefficients than we have. I do not think that the problem you have mentioned is one of the main ones. One of the more difficult things is to get a nice and clean record. Often, the position of the posterior wall or the anterior wall may not be entirely clear-cut and one has the problem of deciding where to draw the line for each of those structures. I think that the relationship of the transverse diameter with the angio has been good and that has been the main thing that we have relied on. If this method proves to be as effective as we think it is, it is quite conceivable that it might offer some advantage over the angiographic technique. After all this has to be obtained from patients who are frightened and who are lying on their backs with tubes in their limbs and with an opaque substance in the arteries which soon disturbs ventricular function. It is therefore conceivable that these methods which can be performed repeatedly in a relaxed patient could have their own standards of excellence which might be quite helpful.

CONCLUDING CHAPTER

SUMMING UP

B. MCA. SAYERS

At the start of this meeting I remarked that it was always difficult to recognize at an early stage those new ideas and concepts that were destined to have a major influence. Before I turn to comment on the potential of some of the powerful new ideas arising from the quantitative approaches about which we have heard, it is interesting to reflect on the situation in the past when new ideas and discoveries came to the surface.

We all know of the remarkable and crucial discoveries of William Harvey about the circulatory system but it is staggering to read what he himself wrote about his most revolutionary discovery – which emerged from his quantitative observations of weight and capacity of the heart.

'What remains to be said upon the quantity and source of the blood' (he wrote). . . 'is of a character so novel and unheard of that I not only fear injury to myself from the envy of a few but I tremble lest I have mankind at large for my enemies, so much doth wont and custom become a second nature.' And as you very well remember he went on to describe how that in the period of an hour the blood put out by the heart would far exceed the weight of a man, and so he came to discuss the concept of a closed loop circulation. How hard it is to really apprehend the iron intellectual constraints that seemed to bind the intellectual processes of the medical and scientific workers of his time. Apparently even Descartes (of all people) welcomed the idea of the circulation of the blood only on the basis of a totally misunderstood view of what Harvey meant. But at least if we are nowadays presented with the skeleton of a wholly new idea or concept the worst that is likely to happen is that we greatly under-value the significance of the matter; on the whole, passions do not tend to run as fiercely as in Harvey's time, ideas are much more a common currency, and we do have regular opportunities for their serious consideration, as in our present meeting, and for coming to terms with their likely importance.

So approaching this meeting objectively, one cannot avoid the realization that quantitation is certainly offering a very wide range of clinically helpful techniques and also that it seems to be generating some powerful general

developments of considerable future importance. And it is worth remember-
ing that for each of the techniques reported here, others exist of which they
are representative, perhaps used for slightly different purposes. Consequently, in surveying the presentations and attempting to evaluate their potential I
need only to emphasize one or two main issues, to select a few of the presentations for special comment, and finally to offer a few general observations,
because, very clearly, there is a heavy weight of solid achievement behind the
techniques and concepts that have been presented.

Perhaps one of the most fascinating developments has come from the
biochemists, with Dr. Hemker's report about the enzyme assay results that
seem to indicate the extent of enzyme leakage from infarcted regions. The
technique depends upon quantitative evaluation, giving results that can be
entered into relatively simple equations that are, in turn, easily solved to give
estimates of the size of the infarct. Since knowledge and the size of infarcted
area, taken together with its location, undoubtedly can provide valuable indications not only for therapy but also in considering the prospects and
planning a regime of rehabilitation, this development is little short of rather
exciting. Who knows – it may even damp down the fires of enthusiasm
amongst those electrocardiographers who believe that estimating infarct size
is very much one of their own preserves?

Another interesting matter is raised in Dr. Schaper's report of his studies in
the development of collateral circulation following coronary artery occlusion. I think many would regard the findings outlined here as a real surprise,
in the speed and extent with which collateral pathways are established, and
this work offers a valuable insight into the factors that determine these
aspects of collateral development. Perhaps not surprisingly, the rate of
coronary artery occlusion is a direct determinant of the result of occlusion,
that is, whether myocardial infarction results or if adequate enlargement of
the collateral system can take place sufficiently rapidly to prevent infarction.
An effective development of the collateral pathways in this case depends
on adequate pre-existing collaterals, as well as on other factors; furthermore,
the growth of the collateral pathway seems to be due to a smooth muscle
mitosis and the rate constant of growth is therefore, not surprisingly, species-
dependent. Nevertheless, despite some of these factors and because of
others, I think we must feel that there are very interesting prospects in this
work; it is not wholly impossible that artificial means of encouraging collateral development may be conceived and this too would be most exciting.

Also on the subject of the occlusion of arteries, and specifically dealing
with arterial occlusive disease, methods of evaluating regional blood flow,

especially by radioactive tracer techniques, have come firmly into the area of clinical application and we have heard of the straight-forward and effective methods that have been developed for use in clinical practice – a classic case of quantitative measurements leading to positive clinical decisions. And so from the hard ground of explicit quantitative measurements to the potentially rewarding but definitely arguable territory of electrocardiography and its quantitative applications.

The key question is this: can the use of electrocardiographic measurements indicate existence, location, and size of an infarcted area? We have had reports, drawing on very careful quantitative measurements, from two groups of workers, presented by Dr. Durrer and Dr. Selvester. To put it succinctly, conclusions differ.

Dr. Durrer is pessimistic. He takes the view, from a position of detailed quantitative experimentation, that while an epicardial electrode (referred to a distant indifferent electrode) can be relied on to give a clear and reliable indication of both magnitude and location of an infarcted region, when the exploring electrode is moved to the thoracic surface, no such reliable indication can be achieved, even in the case of an anteriorly-located infarct. He argues that this is due to the complexity and variability of the electrical conducting pathways to the thoracic surface, and his observations with single leads are persuasive.

The sun shines more brightly in California, and Dr. Selvester is (perhaps for this reason) more optimistic about the prospects. His work is largely based on computer simulations (which themselves stem from detailed electrophysiological studies) and represents an investigation of considerable theoretical and practical sophistication. His team has imagined the entire cardiac muscle mass to be divided into small segments, the depolarization pattern and timing of which is held to be known. Each small segment is then treated as if imbedded in a volume conductor (representing the chest), and contributes electrical current to the computed overall activity (according to its location, size, pattern and timing of depolarization). Dr. Selvester has shown when individual or multiple segments are treated as infarcted, characteristic patterns of the computed electrical activity are found; he has employed a complex quantitative procedure to compute these patterns, taking into account many of the relevant biophysical aspects, and argues that the resulting patterns are useful as reference shapes against which clinical electrocardiograms (in fact vectorcardiograms) can be matched to estimate the location and extent of myocardial damage, from which appropriate therapeutic and rehabilitatory steps can be decided.

There is independent information that allows me to moderate in some measure between these two views, by the expedient of disagreeing very slightly with both. One of the important factors may turn out to be the use of the vector principle; Selvester's work does indeed calculate vector loops, and these require of course at least two leads (several electrodes in most systems) for each planar loop. Inevitably, a system that draws on several electrodes represents a spatial synthesis of the local fluctuations around the thorax, in a way which can be expressed (but not here) in compact and explicit mathematical form. The more the electrodes the more the synthesis, and the precision, and the question then arises: how far is it necessary to go, and what are the penalties of taking insufficient electrode potentials into account?

It happens that I am able to comment on this in some detail; Robert Guardo, working in my own Laboratory, has been able to apply a spatial spectral analysis to the two-dimensional array of electrocardiographic potentials recorded instantaneously over the torso, and from the highest spatial frequency present at any stage in the electrocardiogram, is able to determine the minimum number of sampling points (electrodes) needed to achieve an adequate representation of the distribution of thoracic potentials. Unhappily this number is unrealistically large (probably above 20) for most clinical purposes; this is disturbing, because however reasonable an approximation may be achieved on average by the common, vector, lead systems with many fewer than 20 leads, our findings indicate unequivocally that we must be prepared to encounter, on some occasions, ambiguity in the clinical electrocardiograms, or even, on rarer occasions, a totally misleading representation of the true electrical state. No one has to like this situation but these do appear to be the quantitative facts; they cannot be avoided and should not be overlooked, so it is necessary to accept the implications of a compromise in practically-usable lead systems. So in the present context, the suggestion is that if infarcted myocardial regions do indeed signal their presence by electrical effects altering the pattern of electrical activity distributed over the torso, the full picture of the potential distribution may, in principle, be necessary to characterize the infarct quantitatively and accurately; in practice a limited but substantial number of electrodes is required for the adequate representation of this distribution, and in clinical use, a very much smaller number is feasible, so that precision is limited and reliability by no means complete. Nevertheless, the use of several electrodes, making up a vector lead system, must certainly be more effective, if properly used, than a single exploring lead with one different electrode, in the attempt to represent the exact electrical situation, and thus to seek an accurate indication of the size and location of any infarcted area.

Still on the topic of the electrocardiogram, I should comment on arrhythmia quantitation. Several approaches have been presented, and you will notice an interesting principle now commonly used, that of adaptivity, or learning, as a capability built into the arrythmia measuring apparatus. A suitable waveform is identified and then used as a reference shape to which successive complexes are compared, in order to identify those of abnormal shape. As the wave-shape gradually changes, as always happens with the clinical case, the reference pattern can be adjusted as well to give an adequate representation of the current version of the usual waveform, normal in these circumstances. These ideas have established their value in other areas of signal processing and their use in arrhythmia monitoring devices used for care of the acute patient is both sensible and perhaps overdue. They stem very largely from the work of van Bemmel and his associates on foetal heart monitoring, in which context they have been outstandingly successful.

But I think we do have to be on guard against unwarranted presumptions about the meaning of results obtained from this kind of technique; it is instructive to review the situation briefly. There are two reasons why we are apprehensive about arrhythmias recurring in the acute cardiac patient – one reason commonly mentioned and well-understood, the other less often discussed. The first is that the appearance of certain kinds of arrhythmia, notably due to a ventricular ectopic focus, is a potentially dangerous development because of the risk that the ectopic beat will occur in the so-called vulnerable period of the cardiac cycle, thus greatly increasing the probability that ventricular fibrillation will be initiated. The second reason is the possibility that further damage might be done, for example by the mechanical consequences of arrhythmic beating, in the already debilitated heart. Such effects may be secondary as far as the immediate clinical problem is concerned but we may find that there are significant effects appearing in the long term which should be taken into account, and this does emphasize a need now becoming recognized, to try to evaluate and minimize any potentially deleterious long-term consequences of the choice of clinical therapy. Clearly any such matter would be important in deciding a time for starting, and the extent of, antiarrhythmic therapy, with all its implications, and information about the occurrence of various kinds of arrhythmia would then become vital.

As to the question of arrhythmias of simpler kind acting as precursors of ventricular fibrillation, several factors are involved. Ectopic beats falling in the vulnerable period apparently may initiate fibrillation; so it might be thought that an increase in ectopic frequency would increase the risk of such beats indeed falling in the appropriate perioa of the cardiac cycle. This would be so if the distribution of beats throughout the cardiac cycle were wholly random, or concentrated in certain regions near the vulnerable period, but broadly speaking neither is often true. It is certainly true, in the simplest sense, that the occurrence of a large ectopic rate say, is preceded by a smaller ectopic rate – presumably the rate was initially almost zero. But changes tend to take place in step-wise fashion at irregular times and it seems to be rare for any steady, predictable, trend to appear in the ectopic rate measure; it may then turn out to be unlikely that the frequency of occurrence of any type of arrhythmic beat can be used in coronary care as a guide to anything other than the immediate situation. On the other hand, in view of the consequences of ventricular ectopic arrhythmia in the acute coronary patient, an indication of the imminent onset of this kind of arrhythmia would be useful, and by suitable methods, may be available.

Thus to the fascinating accounts we have had of notable advances in exercise testing by the utilization of quantitative methods. It is clearly sensible to try to normalize the load imposed by an exercise test in order to achieve quantifiable results and provided that a realistic estimate can be made of a patient's expected maximum heart rate, the idea of stressing the patient to some predetermined fraction of this maximum, is a valuable innovation. Dr. Sheffield has based his work on the idea that such a standard stress should generate responses that may have prognostic significance. But it is difficult to find a satisfactory response index, and using as an indicator the extent of electrocardiographic sT segment shifts, usually of ischaemic origin, does have quantitative limitations. Nevertheless, even with this indicator, encouraging results have been achieved, but here again, in order to achieve a reasonable quantitative index on which judgements can be based, detailed quantitative manipulation of the electrocardiographic data is needed. Computer operations are required, not only for quantitative processing of the signals, but also to allow an improved measure of objectivity in reading the results; Sheffield comments, indeed, on the salutory finding of one group of investigators, that observer variability in reading exercise ECG records was a major variable in the attempt at quantitation.

One interesting extension of this technique does warrant more attention than it has received so far; it concerns the use of transient changes of heart rate, rather than steady levels, to standardize the stress, the effects of which are assessed by sT segment shifts. Exercise testing is in itself, of course, basically very sound for reasons now widely accepted. But working with the resulting steady levels, in heart rate and in various electrocardiographic changes, does neglect the important transient compensatory mechanisms which may behave in a fashion more realistically reflecting the capability of the system to cope with stress. A dynamic experiment warrants use of the dynamic quantitative responses that result and I think we are sadly in need of experience along just these lines.

We have been introduced in very lively fashion to the controversy that currently exists between two schools of thought about the behaviour of the heart in shifting blood; one group focusses on the muscular contractile function and the other on the pump function. Now it is clear that there is a relation between the behaviour of a single contractile element and that of the total ventricular chamber in which the single element is embedded. However while extensive and provocative measurements have been achieved for the single element, and Professor Brutsaert has presented a most elegant account of the quantitative experimentation that can be carried out and the instructive conclusions that can be drawn, extrapolation to the total heart muscle is not yet feasible. So the type of studies that Brutsaert reports is restricted at present to the isolated element. However, the isolated element is not an adequate model of the intact heart, and there are several problems in generalizing; one of these is, in a sense, the mechanical analogue of Dr. Selvester's electrocardiographic simulation in embedding an isolated element in a medium of many such elements to determine the overall properties of the total muscle mass. In the mechanical sense it is required to establish the way isolated element properties contribute to overall effects and at present, with a shape as elaborate as that of the heart, this has not been achieved.

Dr. Sandler has presented, very forcefully, the merits of an approach rather different from that of Professor Brutsaert, and draws attention to both haemodynamic and other integrated effects. A basic fact of some importance is that the heart compensates very well in the presence of severe muscle damage, and while this fact does not provide any basis for estimating the residual capability of the heart in the way we would like to see, it does demonstrate the effectiveness of the feedback mechanisms that can be brought into play – mechanisms that are by no means fully understood. As so often happens, there is a real risk for the onlookers to this kind of research that paying detailed attention to the minutiae of one aspect of a physiological system may distract attention from the overall capability and behaviour of the whole system. Perhaps this underlines the growing need for clinicians, as well as basic scientists, to keep their intellectual muscles in good trim to cope with the demands of the growing spectrum of quantitative approaches and above all, the implications of the information they provide.

Well, these matters we have been discussing represent interesting unsolved problems and unresolved differences, but the important fact is that steps are being taken towards intensive quantitative evaluation of overall cardiac function in terms of the elements involved, and their properties; it is undeniable that the better informed the clinician is, about the progress of such investigations, the more fluently will he be able to translate the outcome into clinical practicalities. And equally without doubt, the same goes for the partial insights that emerge as research advances. Indeed, as Professor Hugenholtz has outlined very effectively, many of the clinician's quantitative concepts and ways of thinking about and evaluating cardiac function have been prompted by, and already draw heavily and most usefully on, fundamental ideas arising out of interim findings in basic research. This may look like, in this case, no-man's land between the positions of two schools of thought but it does, in fact, represent a very positive position.

And because it is most essential for the clinician to be able to call upon the interim findings of relevant research in this way it is important that he develop and maintain his skills in the interpretation of research results which are inevitably becoming more quantitative in origin, and more complex in their methods of acquisition. Perhaps it is largely because of the intensively numerical nature of many of the observations involved and because of the manipulations required to translate the primary data into intelligible information, that the computer, in one form or another, is beginning to become an inevitable adjunct to other automatic equipment in the cardiology laboratory, and starting to appear at the bedside in a more-or-less effective role. But – is it welcome?

I think we can recognize two features of the current situation in clinical computing – First, many of the applications are, in terms of computing power, trivial, and merely intended faithfully to duplicate operations of observation, and to some extent judgement, already carried out by skilled staff; second, that by no means all cardiologists would be happy to see the computer appear on their own wards. In view of the unquestionable justice of the former observation (and perhaps because of the latter), criticism of medical computing is common. But what critical opinion often seems to overlook, is that the clinical scientist seeking to introduce and develop computer applications in cardiology, is carrying out something of an act of faith; at the same time, he must, metaphorically, learn to walk before he can run, and in computing terms this means that he must concentrate on gaining experience with procedures of well-understood kind and well-established merit, before branching out into those applications which can utilize computing power sensibly but which inevitably must involve a substantial step into an uncharted region in which the computing science may be complicated and the medical significance initially unknown. Inevitably and correctly the computing clinician must fix his sights on the massive potentiality of the computer, not on his current day-to-day search for experience, but it is most important that the onlooker, his clinical colleague, should not confuse the ongoing search for experience at a relatively primitive level of sophistication and clinical value, with the ultimate possibilities and significance of the computer in clinical cardiology.

The computer is already an important laboratory tool and in this role it has one very special capability – that of operating on virtually any level of complexity at which it is approached. Consequently as demands for quantitative manipulations grow more complex it is feasible to upgrade the demand on the computer. And this particular capability is perhaps at the heart of the potential of the computer at the bed-side, because as methods of communicating with the computer are simplified it will become feasible for all the staff involved with clinical care to make use of the facility at their own level of skill and professional responsibility. If the computer can be supplied with signals from the patient, information about therapy and so on, the nurse can interrogate the computer for certain information, the specialist technician for other information, and the clinician for an overview of the results of quantitatie vprocessing from which, we anticipate, will flow the possibility of more sensitive insight into clinical condition of the patient; perhaps also, as we have seen in some centres already, the computer may be enabled to initiate the therapeutic action indicated to be necessary by its own observations of patient data. All that is lacking in principle is a clear cut idea of what kinds of quantitative processing can profitably be undertaken on the data at the various levels of professional skill and responsibility. This is exactly where the clinician can make an early contribution to the further use of quantitative methods in cardiology. If he is prepared to view sympathetically the efforts of his computing colleagues towards improving and simplifying the way the clinician can use this specialized equipment for optimum clinical purposes, he has taken an important first step to appreciating and understanding the means of great power provided within his grasp for the quantitative evaluation of clinical information. It is greatly to be hoped that a substantial fraction of cardiologists will come forward to advance cardiology in the particular ways opened up by the techniques described in this meeting; and if they do, they will find the computer a vital and fascinating adjunct to their own capabilities.

INDEX OF SUBJECTS